SURGERY IN THE NEW CENTURY

Michael W. Mulholland, M.D, Ph.D.
and Lazar J. Greenfield, M.D.

ISBN 0-9754600-0-5

TABLE OF CONTENTS

CONTRIBUTORS

Juan Arenas, M.D.
Senior Staff Surgeon, Department
of Transplant Surgery, Henry Ford
Hospital, Detroit, MI

Darrell A. Campbell, Jr., M.D.
Henry King Ransom Professor of
Surgery and Chief of Clinical Affairs,
University of Michigan, Ann Arbor, MI

Alfred E. Chang, M.D.
Professor, Section of General Surgery,
Department of Surgery, University of
Michigan, Ann Arbor, MI

Lisa M.Colletti, M.D.
Associate Professor, Section of General
Surgery, Department of Surgery, and
Associate Dean, Medical School,
University of Michigan, Ann Arbor, MI

Matthew J. Eagleton, M.D.
Assistant Professor, Section of Vascular
Surgery, Department of Surgery,
University of Michigan, Ann Arbor, MI

J. Roland Folse, M.D.
Emeritus Professor, Department of
Surgery, Southern Illinois University
School of Medicine

Andrew A. Freiberg, M.D.
Assistant Professor of Orthopedic
Surgery, Massachusetts General
Hospital, Harvard Medical School,
Boston, MA

Paul G. Gauger, M.D.
Assistant Professor, Section of General
Surgery, Department of Surgery,
University of Michigan, Ann Arbor, MI

Lazar J. Greenfield, M.D.
Professor and Chair Emeritus,
Department of Surgery, University of
Michigan, Ann Arbor, MI

Ronald B. Hirschl, M.D.
Professor, Section of Pediatric Surgery,
Department of Surgery, University of
Michigan, Ann Arbor, MI

Mark D. Iannettoni, M.D., M.B.A.
Johann L. Ehrenhaft Professor
and Chairman, Department of
Cardiothoracic Surgery, University of
Iowa Hospitals and Clinics, Roy and
Lucille Carver College of Medicine,
Iowa City, IA

William M. Kuzon, Jr., M.D., Ph.D.
Professor and Head, Section of Plastic
Surgery, Department of Surgery and
Research Associate Professor, Institute
of Gerontology, University of Michigan,
Ann Arbor, MI

Jenny J. Mace
Senior Staff Assistant, Department of
Anesthesiology, University of Michigan,
Ann Arbor, MI

Michael W. Mulholland, M.D., Ph.D.
Frederick A. Coller Distinguished
Professor and Chair, Department of
Surgery, University of Michigan, Ann
Arbor, MI

Michael O'Reilly, M.D., M.S.
Clinical Associate Professor, Department
of Anesthesiology, University of
Michigan, Ann Arbor, MI

Richard N. Pierson, III, M.D.
Associate Professor of Surgery,
Department of Cardiothoracic Surgery,
Vanderbilt University Medical Center,
Nashville, TN

Jeffrey D. Punch, M.D.
Associate Professor, Section of General
Surgery, Department of Surgery,
University of Michigan, Ann Arbor, MI

Michael S. Sabel, M.D.
Assistant Professor, Section of General
Surgery, Department of Surgery,
University of Michigan, Ann Arbor, MI

Frank G. Scholl, M.D.
Resident in Cardiothoracic Surgery,
Vanderbilt University Medical Center,
Nashville, TN

Bruce C. Steffes, M.D.
Retired general surgeon and missionary,
World Medical Mission

Paul A. Taheri, M.D., M.B.A.
Associate Professor of Surgery, Associate
Dean, Medical School, and Assistant
Research Scientist, School of Business
Administration, University of Michigan,
Ann Arbor, MI

Kevin K. Tremper, M.D., Ph.D.
Professor and Chair, Department of
Anesthesiology, University of Michigan,
Ann Arbor, MI

Gilbert R. Upchurch, Jr., M.D.
Assistant Professor, Section of Vascular
Surgery, Department of Surgery,
University of Michigan, Ann Arbor, MI

Edwin G. Wilkins, M.D.
Associate Professor, Section of Plastic
Surgery, Department of Surgery,
University of Michigan, Ann Arbor, MI

J. Stuart Wolf, Jr., M.D.
Associate Professor, Department of
Urology, University of Michigan, Ann
Arbor, Michigan

Chapter 1

THE CHANGING SURGICAL PATIENT

MICHAEL W. MULHOLLAND, M.D., Ph.D.

As surgeons anticipate the provision of care in the future, the changing nature of the surgical patient is a first consideration. The population of the United States is increasing due to greater life expectancy and the effects of immigration; population growth will be compounded by other factors, including internal population shifts. On average, surgical patients in the future will be older. Surgical procedures will be offered to patients increasingly at the extremes of life, and in the case of fetal surgery, before birth. The social fabric of the United States will also change, with significant demographic shifts occurring due to differential birth rates and changing patterns of immigration. Surgical care will be rendered in an environment that is socially, economically, and scientifically different than that experienced at the turn of the 21st century. An appreciation of the changing nature of American society will be important to inform decisions regarding the delivery of health services in the future.

The United States Census Bureau marked its 100th year of service in 2000. The Census Bureau provides data from surveys, administrative records, and censuses to government officials and policymakers.(1) Health care providers must also use this agency for the highest quality data in planning for future health care delivery.

At the beginning of the 21st century, the resident population of the United States was estimated to be 273 million, a 10% increase relative to 1990. Not all population segments of the American population have grown at the same rate, however. Population growth has been most rapid for Asian, Pacific Islander, and Hispanic populations, fueled by both nativity and migration from abroad. African American and American Indian populations have also experienced rapid population growth. In contrast, the population growth for Whites who were not of Hispanic origin was only 4%. The White non-Hispanic share of the total population in 2000 had decreased to 72% from 76% a decade previously. The Asian and Pacific Islander populations now account for 4% of the American total, numbering 11 million residents in 2000. Hispanic residents account for 12% of the American population, with the African American population numbering 35 million, a 13% share of the total.

At the beginning of the 20th century, American women could expect to give birth to 4 children during their reproductive years. This fertility rate remained constant until the end of World War II but had gradually declined to 1.8 children by the mid 1970's. Without major fluctuation, overall American fertility rates remained at approximately 2 births per woman for the past 20 years. A rate of 2 births per woman is below the long-term replacement level. However, childbearing patterns differ greatly among racial and ethnic groups within the United States. Among Hispanic women, the average number of births during childbearing years approximates 2.4. The fertility rate among African American, Asian, and Pacific Islander women in the United States is intermediate at 2.1 births per woman. White non-Hispanic women have a significantly lower fertility level, averaging 1.8 births each.

The southern and western regions of the United States have experienced the highest average growth rates, while midwestern and northeastern states have lagged behind. In the decade before 2000, the southern regions grew by 13% while the western population increased by 16%. Over the same 10 years, the population of the Midwest region increased by 6%, while the increment in population in the northeast was only 2%. The United States is increasingly suburban. In all areas of the country, population growth has been most rapid in suburban areas. By 2000, 62% of Americans lived in metropolitan areas outside of the central cities. This tread is expected to continue. Americans continue to be extremely mobile. Approximately 40 million people, 16% of the total population, can be expected to move within the United States in each calendar year.

The Census Bureau projects that over the next 25 years net population change, expressed as number of births minus deaths plus net migration, will be greatest in three states, California, Texas, and Florida.(2) The population of each of these states is projected to increase by more than 6 million persons by the year 2025. By that time, population changes in these three states alone will account for more than 45% of the net change in the United States. California, currently the most populus state, is expected to account for 15% of the United States population by 2025. The net increase in population, estimated at 18 million people, is nearly the population of New York State in 2000.

The United States is becoming a more culturally diverse nation. A significant driving force in this change is continuing immigration from other countries.(3) In 2000, approximately 30 million foreign born individuals lived in the United States, representing 11% of the total population. Among the foreign born population, half were from Latin America, 25% were born in Asia, and 15% were from Europe. The remainder was derived from other portions of the globe. Most of the immigration to this country has occurred in the western states with approximately 40% of new arrivals. Smaller percentages have moved to the south and to the northeast, with the smallest percentage, only 11%, in the Midwest. The households of foreign-born Americans are significantly larger than those of native born. In 2000, 27% of households in which a foreign born person was the householder consist of 5 or more people. Only 13% of households of native born individuals were this large.

The American population will age significantly in the next 20 years.(4) At the beginning of the 21st century, half of all people living in the United States were age

36 or older. This median age increased by 3 years relative to 1990. Young persons, defined by the Census Bureau as newborns to age 19, are projected to account for a smaller proportion of the population and in 2025, 27% relative to 29% in 1995. As the baby boom generation (those born between 1946 and 1964) reaches retirement age, the size and proportion of the elderly population is predicted to increase in all states. In 2000, approximately 25 million American men and 31 million American women were age 55 and older. The male to female ratio was 8 to 10 for older Americans.

At the beginning of the 20th century, life expectancy in the United States was 47 years. By the year 2000, life expectancy had increased to 74 years for men and 79 for women. The Census Bureau estimates that the growth in elderly population in the years 2000 to 2010 will be modest, but that the elderly population will increase rapidly in the period of 2010 through 2030, due to the influx of the baby boom generation into this age group. By 2020 it is estimated that more than 7 million individuals will be older than 85 years. Internal migration will shift elderly populations increasingly to states in the south and west from the northeast and midwestern regions.

The increasingly elderly population will have very significant impact upon the health care delivery system. The incidence of disability increases as a function of age. Among those aged 45-54 years, approximately one-fourth has some form of disability, with 14% reported severe disability. For individuals aged 80 and older, 74% report some disability, 58% severe disability. Fully 35% of individuals in this age group require some level of personal assistance secondary to this disability. However, poor health is not universal among the elderly. The Census Bureau reports that among non-institutionalized persons in 1992, 75% aged 65 –74 considered their health to be good, very good, or excellent.

The economics of health care delivery, particularly health insurance coverage, will be a major issue in the foreseeable future.(5) In 1999, 16% of the American population was without health insurance coverage for the entire year, amounting to almost 43 million individuals. Employment-based private health insurance is the most important means of coverage in the United States; 63% of Americans receive health care benefits through this mechanism. Nearly one-fourth of the American population is currently covered by a government health plan, including Medicare at 13%, Medicaid at 10%, and military health insurance plans at 3%. Coverage by medical insurance is closely related by both economic and social factors. For Americans below the poverty line, the uninsured rate approximates 30%. Insured rates for White non-Hispanic Americans is good at 90%. Coverage rates for African American, Asian, and Pacific Islander Americans are similar to that for White, non-Hispanics, approximating 82%. The coverage rate among Hispanic Americans is the lowest at 68%. Among all ethnic groups, the likelihood of insurance coverage increases as the level of education rises. Insurance coverage also reflects income levels.

For households with an annual income of $75,000, only 8% of people are without insurance coverage. For households with incomes with less than $25,000, 24% of individuals are not covered.

While the economics of health care delivery 20 years hence are impossible to predict with accuracy, several trends appear likely to continue. An increasingly elderly population, with high frequency of co-morbidities, will be cared for in an increasingly ambulatory environment. Outpatient surgery, now amounting to almost 30% of operative case loads, seems certain to grow in the next two decades. This trend will create a dichotomy of increasing inpatient acuity and greater volumes of outpatient procedures. Outpatient support systems will need to grow proportionately to care for these patients.

Personalized Biology

Changing demographics will create a different patient base for surgeons in the 21st century. The revolution in molecular biology, in imaging, and in biocomputation will provide surgeons with increasingly sophisticated, highly personalized information about their patients that will influence surgical care to an even greater extent. Surgical advances in the 20th century were based upon a dramatic and unprecedented understanding of surgical physiology and anatomy. Development of anesthetic techniques, surgical instrumentation, and physiological monitoring permitted the introduction of very invasive procedures performed through large open incisions.(6) The surgery of the 21st century will be based upon advances in genetics and molecular biology, improved medical imaging, advances in information technology and in minimally invasive surgical techniques and instrumentation. Surgical care is entering a period of revolutionary change.

Personalized Genomics

The scientific effort to sequence the human genome, spearheaded by the National Institutes of Health, has become one of the most significant advances in medicine as we enter the new century. A preliminary map of the human genome DNA sequence was provided in 2001. A more complete and more accurate reference sequence is expected by the year 2003. Currently, it is estimated that between 40,000 and 100,000 human genes exist. This milestone achievement provides a framework for the subsequent, thorough exploration of the human genetic code. A full understanding of genetic determinants of human health and disease will require an understanding of this entire set of genes and of the proteins whose expression they direct. The work will occupy medical scientists, including surgeons, for the next several decades.

There are a number of technologies which can be utilized to define gene expression and to profile gene activation in particular cell types or tissues. Current techniques include differential screening of cDNA libraries, subtraction cDNA hybridization, differential display of RNA and traditional methods of gene expression and sequencing. Recently, DNA microarrays had provided an effective way of examining minute samples for the expression of thousands of genes simultaneously.(7)

A DNA microarray, or gene chip, consists of ordered DNA molecules of known sequence placed on a solid surface. A description of DNA microarrays as a high capacity system to monitor RNA levels was first provided by Brown and colleagues in 1995. First developed to examine up to 1,000 genes simultaneously, improvements in current techniques will soon permit the examination of the total number of human genes (approximately 50,000) in a single experiment.

For cDNA arrays, nucleic acid fragments of known sequence are placed robotically as micro spots.(8) Typically substrate-coded glass slides are used, creating a precise two-dimensional array of known sequence. The oligonucleotides attached to these slides represent the target of the assay to which an unknown mixture of complimentary DNAs (cDNAs) attaches. The cDNA derived from the sample is usually fluorescently labeled. Currently, a two-color scheme is utilized. Image processing programs has been developed to detect the micro spots and to quantify them. The fluorescent intensity of each spot corresponds to the relative cDNA abundance present in the sample.

This general approach permits evaluation of gene expression patterns among thousands of defined genes.(9, 10) Vast amounts of data are generated, and specialized computational software has been developed to direct analysis. At the current state of development, most microarray studies have been retrospective surveys attempting to detect general patterns of gene expression. This approach has been employed extensively in oncology to describe transcriptional patterns in common cancer types, for example, colon cancer or breast cancer.

To reach its full clinical potential, microarray analysis must meet three criteria: 1) analysis must be conducted real-time rather than retrospectively; 2) analysis must be applied to individual patients; and 3) the functional roles of the entire human genome must be defined. In the near future, it will be possible to sequence the genome of each individual patient from a sample obtained by phlebotomy. A series of personalized oligonucleotides can then be created corresponding to each gene. Using a modified microarray process, analogous to that outlined above, it will be possible to determine each individual patient's reactions to physiological stresses or response to therapies or drug exposures.

Using current technology, an extensive literature has developed describing metabolic changes attending exposure to drugs. Microarray analysis could predict individual patient responsiveness to drugs and may also help to unravel underlying molecular mechanisms on an individual basis. This technology will permit appropriate monitoring of potential toxicities and modification of drug doses in individual patients.

Physiologic states and disease processes may also be examined as to their biological impact in individual patients. A good example is the cellular response to bacterial endotoxins. Lipopolysaccharide is formed by Gram negative bacteria, and is a major contributor to the septic state attending Gram negative bacteriemia. Microarray systems have demonstrated that approximately 4,000 genes are differentially regulated in animals after exposure to lipopolysaccharide. In the future, this analysis will be translated to individual patients in response to sepsis, and other specific challenges. The impact of nutritional status has been examined in animal models using DNA microarray technology. The changes that occur with altered nutrition in human subjects can also be examined in detail in the future using this approach.

Personalized Proteomics

Progress on the sequencing phase of the human genome project has now focused attention on an even more important topic than gene transcription, the function of the corresponding proteins that these genes encode. Gene sequencing information has been complemented by recent advances in molecular and structural biology to determine three-dimensional protein structures. The three dimensional structural information provides clues as to particular protein functions. Currently, is it estimated that less than 30% of all human proteins have a known function.

Microarray technologies can also be used as high throughput devices to examine protein function.(11) These microarray devices are constructed by covalently attaching proteins to microscope glass slides. The methodology is similar to that used to produce gene chips, employing robotic printing of the array and imaging scanners for detection. At the spotting density used for most studies, it is possible to examine more than 10,000 samples in the area of a standard microscopic slide (2.5 cm x 7.5 cm). In addition, examination for protein-protein interactions, identification of substrate for enzymes, and screening for small molecule-protein interactions are possible. These miniaturized formats permit one to examine samples in a highly compressed assay. In theory, it will soon be possible to study every protein in a specific cell type, organized tissue, or whole organism.(12, 13)

Cellular Microarrays

Genes are not transcribed and proteins are not normally expressed in a cell-free environment. The context of the cellular expression has significant influence on both of these processes, as they in turn influence cellular function. A recently described technique permits a microarray-type examination of cells expressing defined cDNAs.(14) The strategy permits a high throughput analysis of gene function in mammalian cells. A living microarray can be constructed of cell clusters expressing defined gene products. These cell clusters can then be assayed for any property detectable on their surface.

To create these microarrays, defined DNAs are plated on glass cover slides using a robotic arrayer. After drying, the DNA spots are exposed to a lipid transfection reagent. The spots are then covered by a layer of adherent mammalian cells in culture. Cells contacting the attached plasmid DNA become transfected and specifically express the gene in question and its resulting protein.

Transfected cell microarrays have advantage over microarrays strategies using only cDNA or even proteins. The cDNAs are not isolated from the cells demonstrating phenotype of interest and the signal is concentrated in a small area so that expression increases of small magnitude can be detected.(14) Transfected cell microarrays can be used to screen live cells, allowing the detection of transient changes. The microarrays of DNA are stable for months and can be converted into mammalian cell cultures when needed. Surgeons in the future will employ cellular microarrays when their patients undergo specific physiological challenges or are confronted by defined disease dates.

With currently available technology, it is possible to achieve densities of up to 10,000 cell clusters on a standard microscope slide. According to a recent report, at these densities, the entire set of human genes could be examined on a small number of slides.(14)

Stem Cells

Bone marrow stem cells are capable of self-renewal, and under the proper conditions, can differentiate into either hematopoietic or epithelial cell lines. Recent investigations in animals and in humans have shown that mesenchymal stem cells have the potential to differentiate into bone marrow, fat, cartilage, bone, tendon, or muscle. Human blood contains stem cells that can differentiate into cells, which are indistinguishable from those of the native liver, skin, or gastrointestinal tract.(15) The ability of stem cells to differentiate functionally and to act as liver, skin, or intestinal epithelium is currently unknown, however.

Surgeons in the future will be able to access stem cells by phlebotomy. In addition to potential for functional organ replacement, stem cells may also be used in the future for diagnostic purposes. Stem cells derived from circulating blood will be induced, under proper in vitro conditions, to differentiate into hepatocytes, skin cells, or intestinal epithelial cells as desired. Used in an assay system analogous to cellular microarrays, functionality under surgical disease states could be tested.(16) For example, the effect of fasting, or hypovolemia or sepsis could be modeled in vitro and individual responses predicted before patients were exposed to these stresses. Susceptibility to drug toxicity or to undesired secondary effects of other agents could be predicted without exposing the patient to the potentially harmful therapy.

Personalized Bioengineering

Bioengineers, clinicians, and biologists have combined their talents to design replacements for the human body. This goal has captured the imagination of the public, most vividly with the implantation of total artificial hearts into patients with end-stage heart disease.(17) Replacements for human organs in development and in application span virtually all systems from blood to tendons to vision to joints.(18-20) Most efforts have focused upon developing off-the-shelf prostheses and replacements for human bodily function. Future efforts will be directed at individualizing these devices and biotechniques for specific patients.

Personalized Medical Imaging

Cross sectional anatomic imaging, pioneered approximately two decades ago has revolutionized the practice of medicine. Conventional axial imaging techniques include ultrasound, computed tomography and magnetic resonance imaging. These techniques permit surgeons to detect anatomic detail in normal organs and anatomical changes associated with disease. These modalities do not provide information on organ function or on metabolic derangements associated with disease. To date, functional imaging has been represented by nuclear medical techniques, and is exemplified by positron emission tomography (PET scanning).

Structural and functional imagings are increasingly viewed as complimentary modalities. The ability to merge biological function with detailed structural anatomy will affect a second revolution in medical practice.

This merging requires the fusion of two imaging methods, referred to as image registration.(21) Registration requires that the center of the volume imaged by one method be matched to the center of volume imaged by the second method. Registration also orients slice planes and the size of one image to the other. Earliest efforts at registration used external markers, which were visible on each imaging method to assure the spatial coordinates were accurately aligned.

In the future, image registration will more likely be achieved by having the two involved scanners calibrated to one another. To achieve this integration, the scanners must be brought to the same physical location, and the technique assumes that the patient remains motionless between image acquisitions. Devices are currently operational which permit sequential acquisition of both anatomic and functional data by combining computed tomography (transmission) and positron image tomography (PET emission). Having a single scanner with both capabilities reduces potential sources of error that can be caused by positioning and movement, and eliminates the requirement for external markers or complicated mathematic formulae.

Proven imaging agents, which rely upon physiologic function, are also becoming available. An example is fluorodeoxyglucose (FDG), a glucose analog which is differentially taken up by malignant cells. Foci of abnormally increased FDG uptake are considered suggestive of malignant tissue. Metabolic changes often predate morphologic changes associated with disease, as detected by conventional CT scanning. Combined PET/CT scanning with FDG has been demonstrated to detect deposits of cancer cells before they became large enough to cause anatomic distortion.(22-24)

In the future it should be possible to obtain whole body imaging with simultaneous acquisition of multiple kinds of information. One can imagine simultaneous mammography, virtual colonoscopy, brain scan, and examination of liver. In the future, these examinations may be performed as screens, in the absence of symptoms or disease, and repetitively. In this way, a personalized record through time of both physical and structural changes could be obtained for patients.

Personalized Biocomputation

Human beings are complex organisms, populated by billions of cells, each containing billions of molecules and expressing perhaps 50,000 genes in a variable manner. To understand biological phenomenon in the future, surgeons will need to document and analyze molecular compositions and interactions within cells. To do so will require new methods of biocomputation, greatly exceeding currently available analytical capacity.

Currently under development are mathematical models of entire systems that use cellular and molecular models as building blocks for integrated understanding. Powerful computers and graphic interfaces have made possible the development of complicated models that span levels of integration from gene to organ systems to the entire organism. To convert massive volumes of raw data would currently overwhelm most desktop machines and even powerful super computers. Through connectivity across the Internet, large numbers of personal computers may be entrained to cooperate and share capacity for huge computing tasks.

Current efforts to integrate electrical, mechanical, and optical systems on a microscopic scale with micro fluidic systems have been combined with bioinformatics.(26) These approaches may presage the development of a "lab on a chip" enabling analysis of thousands of molecules simultaneously from a single sample. This may also permit surgeons to simulate reality without exposing their patients to potentially dangerous conditions.

Integration of technologies in the future will permit powerful new synergies. Personalized molecular biology, personalized imaging, and personalized biocomputation will be integrated and become portable in the form of implantable cybernetics. The full use of these technologies will require surgeons of the future to be familiar with more than just the use of a scalpel.

REFERENCES

1. U.S. Census Bureau. Population profile of the United States. Current population reports 1999; Series P23-205.

2. U.S. Census Bureau. Population projections: States, 1995-2025. Current population reports 1997; Series P25-1131.

3. U.S. Census Bureau. The foreign-born population in the United States. Current population reports 2001; Series P20-534.

4. U.S. Census Bureau. The older population in the United States. Current population reports 2000; Series P20-532.

5. U.S. Census Bureau. Health insurance coverage. Current population reports 2001; Series P60-215.

6. Brunicardi FC. Molecular surgery and biology. Am J Surg 2000; 180:397-401.

7. Watson SJ, Meng F, Thompson RC, Akil H. The "chip" as a specific genetic tool. Biol Psychiatry 2000; 48:1147-1156.

8. Arcellana-Panlilio M, Robbins SM. Global gene expression profiling using DNA microarrays. Am J Gastro Liver Physiol 2002; 282: G397-G402, 2002.

9. Zapico MEF, Ahmad US, Urrutia R. DNA microarrays: Revolutionary insight into the living genome. Surgery 2001; 130(3):403-407.

10. Hernandez A, Evers BM. Functional genomics: clinical effect and the evolving role of the surgeon. Arch Surg 1999; 134(11):1209-1215.

11. Haab BB, Dunham MJ, Brown PO. Protein microarrays for highly parallel detection and quantitation of specific proteins and antibodies in complex solutions. Genome Biol 2001;2(2):1-13.

12. Feng H. A protein microarray. Nature Structural Biol 2000; 7(10):829.

13. Christendat D, Yee A, Dharamsi A, et al. Structural proteomics of an archaeon. Nature Structural Biol 2000; 79(10):903-909.

14. Zlauddin J, Sabatini DM. Microarrays of cells expressing defined cDNAs. Nature 2001; 441:107-110.

15. Körbling M, Katz RL, Khanna MA, et al. Hepatocytes and epithelial cells of donor organ in receipients of peripheral-blood stem cells. N Engl J Med 2002;346(10): 738-746.

16. Kelly DL, Rizzino A. DNA microarray analyses of genes regulated during the differentiation of embryonic stem cells. Molec Reprod Develop 2000;56:113-123.

17. McCarthy PM, Smith WA. Mechanical circulatory support-a long and winding road. Science 2002;295:998-999.

18. Squires JE. Artifical blood. Science 2002;295:1002-1005.

19. Pennisi E. Tending tender tendons. Science 2002;295:1011.

20. Zrenner E. Will retinal implants restore vision? Science 2002;295:10221025.

21. Shreve PD. Adding structure to function. J Nucl Med 2000;41(8):1380-1382.

22. Beyer T, Townsend DW, Brun T, et al. A combined PET/CT scanner for clinical oncology. J Nucl Med 2000;41(8):1369-1379.

23. Israel O, Keidar Z, Losilevsky G, et al. The fusion of anatomic and physiologic imaging in the management of patients with cancer. Sem Nucl Med 2001;31(3):191-205.

24. Ketai L, Hartshorne M. Potential uses of computed tomography-SPECT and computed tomography-coincidence fusion images of the chest. Clin Nucl Med 2001;26:433-441.

25. Rew DA. Modelling in surgical oncology-Part III: Massive data sets and complex systems. Eur J Surg Oncology 2000;26:805-809.

26. Griffith LG, Grodzinsky AJ. Advances in biomedical engineering. JAMA 2001;285(5):556-561.

Chapter 2

THE CHANGING SURGEON

DARRELL A. CAMPBELL, JR., M.D.

The surgeon of the future will be a product of the past. This is to say that contemporary surgeons must identify critical problems in the field and respond positively. While other parts of this collection of essays on surgery in the 21st century will focus on technical or biological advances, here two different but important areas for advancement are discussed: how the surgeon as a person relates to the discipline of surgery, and how the discipline of surgery relates to society.

The Surgeon and the Discipline of Surgery

There are two important issues that involve the relationship between the individual surgeon and the discipline of surgery. Dramatic change in both areas is critical to the health of the profession. First, we must learn how to reconcile the conflict between commitment (hard work) and comfort (lifestyle) if we are to attract the most competent and capable trainees. Second, we must understand what factors lead established surgeons to become detached from the profession, manifest by declining membership in professional societies, or to retire entirely from surgery at an early age. This is perhaps the most costly of all problems facing surgery and society. As a corollary, we must understand how some surgeons become "engaged" with work, and manage to derive immense satisfaction from the discipline, while also experiencing a balanced, happy life.

The lifestyle of a surgeon has always been difficult. Still, a sufficient number of students have entered the field. Presumably in the past, the difficulties lumped in the "lifestyle" category of problems were considered to be more than offset by the rewards of the discipline. This balance has shifted; fewer students enter the more demanding areas of surgery, and of those that do choose surgery, an alarming number change direction midway through training.(1) Thus, either the perceived "cost" of a surgical career to the student, usually seen in terms of family or personal development, has increased, or the perceived benefit from the field, in terms of personal satisfaction, has decreased. Whatever the reason, students are staying away in droves.

Likewise, it is important to consider the fate of the actively practicing surgeon. One has only to sit in the locker room of any operating room to get a sense of the general level of frustration and stress that is the daily routine. This dissatisfaction seems to have increased in recent years. Previous data has demonstrated the sequelae of stress for the active surgeon, such as increased rates of suicide (2), marital discord

(3), and substance abuse.(4) Detailed psychological testing has shown higher rates of free floating and hysterical anxiety (5) among surgeons than other medical practitioners. Reliable data on the rate of attrition from surgery of established surgeons is hard to come by, but more and more anecdotal cases have arisen in which mid-career surgeon has either changed medical specialties or retired early. A variety of explanations are usually offered, but the inescapable conclusion must be drawn that, at its root, the problem lies in an inability of the surgeon to tolerate the stress of the modern surgical environment.

Although it is difficult to prove, a reasonable hypothesis is that unrecognized stress underlies the day to day difficulties surgeons face. If this is true, there are strategies that can be adopted which will address this point, albeit over a period of many years. Many such strategies have been enacted in non-medical organizations, with remarkable results, and yet organized medicine, and particularly surgery, has been resistant to this type of approach. Surgeons are above this level of vulnerability, so it is thought. The process is insidious, is hard to recognize, but real. Pilots, one of the professional groups most akin to surgeons, have recognized that stress affects performance, and have adopted stress reduction strategies, most prominently in the area of workload reduction. Pilots also are faced with stressful situations, and shoulder great responsibility. Although the analogy has its limits, what has worked for them should work for us.

Why are we unable to tolerate high levels of stress? Certainly, biological factors play a role in conferring resistance or vulnerability. In the psychological literature, this is referred to as "hardiness".(6) This is another way of saying that stress is a relative term; what is very stressful to one may not be stressful to another. And yet when the profession is considered in its entirety, the sequelae of stress are more prominent among surgeons than other non-medical professionals. Assuming a normal distribution of the hardiness characteristic in surgeons, this would suggest that stress intolerance relates to the higher level of stress experienced in the surgical workplace. The next time a clamp slips off the vena cava try to argue that this is not the case.

If stress is inherently high in surgery, and has important consequences, what do we do to increase our resistance? This is where we as a profession have fallen down and need to devise a strategy. The strategy must involve the surgical training period because this is where impressionable young trainees have gotten off course. Krizek has recently written on this subject, and indicated 10 factors associated with the educational process which he considers "impairing", i.e. lead to problems in later life for the practicing surgeon.(7) Prominent among the impairing factors are long work hours, emotional burden, and the propensity for mistakes. The focus on work ethic at the expense of balance is a serious deficiency. Importantly, the lack of recognition of stress in the training process, and lack of instruction in established stress reduction techniques sews the seeds for the problems which we face today.

One approach for the problem of stress in surgery is to pick a reliable measure of stress, assess the measure in the current population of surgeons, and evaluate stress reduction strategies against this parameter. But what parameter would be best for this purpose? One possibility is the psychological construct of burnout. Burnout is defined as "emotional exhaustion, depersonalization and reduced personal accomplishment that can occur among individuals who work with people in some capacity".(8) As it is thought to result from repetitive stressful interactions, certainly an apt description of a surgical practice, this way of characterizing stress in surgery has some appeal. Importantly, the burnout phenomenon is something that is measurable, using a well-validated survey instrument, the Maslach Burnout Inventory.(8)

When we applied the Maslach Burnout Inventory to 582 actively practicing American surgeons, we got a snapshot of the level of burnout experienced by practitioners working on the front lines.(9) At the same time, we gained information about what drives the successful, "engaged" surgeon. There are a few important insights that were gained from this analysis. First, 32% of respondents were seen to have "high" levels of emotional exhaustion, measured on a national scale drawn from many thousands of individuals. Whether this represents a crisis to our profession is open to debate, but most patients wouldn't want to undergo surgery by a surgeon feeling this way, having "nothing left to give", a feeling which characterizes this state. Thirteen percent scored high in levels of detachment, the second phase of the process, which is germane to the problems of our deteriorating doctor-patient relations. Doctors in the "high" level of this category tend to view patients as inanimate objects, or worse, as deserving of their problems. These feelings were not related to practice setting (academic, private or mixed), indicating underlying factors deeper than those that are commonly pinpointed.

	Type of Practice		
	Private Practice (n = 163)	Full-Time Academic (n = 186)	Private Practice with Academic Affiliation (n = 190)
High Emotional Exhaustion	29%	31%	33%
High Depersonalization	14%	9%	19%
Low Personal Accomplishment	5%	4%	4%

We as a profession should be alarmed by this data and take steps to address the underlying issues. But these data should also serve as a baseline, and the profession should monitor the results on a regular basis to evaluate any interventions taken. Approximately the same percentage of surgeons were seen to be "engaged" with work, which is to say that they had low levels of exhaustion and detachment, and high levels of personal accomplishment. Our profession needs to understand what leads to the latter category, so that we can emphasize and encourage development of these factors in training. A reasonable workload, balance, and a sense of "meaning" from work were found to be particularly important.

We also found that the burnout condition was more a function of the younger rather than the older surgeon. This finding points to the importance of preparing our trainees for the real surgical world, with all its problems, during the residency period. In the current surgical training culture, a significant proportion seems to "burnout" soon after leaving the training environment. It seems achievable that we can reverse this tendency by attending to those issues during training.

One of the most significant issues associated with the burnout condition was found to be balance, or rather the lack of it, in surgeons scoring high in burnout.

	Burnout Subscales	
Supplemental Questionnaire	**Emotional Exhaustion**	**Depersonalization**
Workload is overwhelming?	0.61**	0.28**
Have achieved balance between work, family and personal growth?	-0.56**	-0.31**
Time for personal growth and development?	-0.42**	-0.20**
Career expectations met?	-0.42**	-0.30**
Autonomy and decision involvement?	-0.39**	-0.18**
Work gives sense of meaning?	-0.26**	-0.30**

**Correlation is significant at the 0.01 level (2-tailed)

Specifically, when asked the question "have you achieved balance between work, family and personal growth", a very high correlation was noted between the burnout condition and a "no" answer to this question. As mentioned before, the data targeted the younger surgeons. Two other important correlations identified a failure of career expectations to be met, and a lack of a sense of "meaning" from the surgical career in the burnout category. What comes into focus from this data is the picture of a disillusioned young surgeon who seeks more balance in his life and more meaning from his surgical practice.

To address these problems the surgeon of the 21st century must look inward. We have not been good at this. It has been too easy to drift into the overwork category, which leads to imbalance, family frustrations, and detachment or even cynicism to patients. As a result, the sense of mission is lost. A sense of mission or purpose has traditionally been the great antidote to burnout. Mother Teresa was never in the burnout category.

Surgical training programs of the 21st century must facilitate change. An emphasis must be placed on achieving balance. This can be done by giving a more prominent role to surgeons who have achieved balance, and asking them to teach residents about this important goal.

How did they balance their lives? What gave them satisfaction? How were roadblocks over come? The answers to these questions are as important to a surgeon as technical experience. A career in surgery is more than operating; it also involves adjustment to a challenging lifestyle. This can be taught just as operative procedures are taught. The current push for limitation of surgical work hours will help. Respondents in the burnout category indicated rather dramatically that they felt work was "overwhelming". This habit of taking on too much was probably initiated during residency, and learned from prominent professors.

Professionalism and mission are two areas that deserve more exposure in the residency; electives in underserved areas might be a good beginning and involvement in surgical societies open to residents should be encouraged. Each resident should be asked to keep a record of notes from grateful patients and regular discussions of these inspirational cases should occur. This will help impressionable young surgeons remember why they went into surgery. Classes in stress reduction should be mandatory. In such classes areas covered are personal management skills, including prioritization, setting goals and time management. Relationship skills are covered, including friendships, assertiveness, and outlook skills involving creativity and sense of humor are practiced. Stamina skills are also emphasized, involving exercise, relaxation and nutrition. When used in a medical training program, such a program was successful in reducing stress measured objectively.(10) Other programs may focus on the common non-clinical problems encountered by residents including "interactions with nurses", "difficult patient", "management of medical mistakes", "physician-physician interaction" and many others.(11) The discussion and insight into these areas pinpoints stress that can be avoided, as it builds on experience and avoids reinventing the wheel with each new class of residents.

Finally, and probably most importantly, the families of the trainees need to be more fully integrated into the program. Discussion groups including spouses are helpful and often yield creative suggestions for time management or stress reduction. All of this is to say that a perceived change in direction and emphasis during residency will set the stage for the surgeon of the 21st century. This surgeon will be more open to the concept that stress influences performance, that surgeons may find a stress point beyond which they do not function well, and that with some attention to human frailties during training, the long distance race which is a surgical career, is likely to be finished rather than derailed.

The Discipline of Surgery and Society

If the individual surgeon should look inward to make the transition to the 21st century, it is also true that society has begun to examine the discipline of surgery more closely. Society expects quality, and a way to measure it. The old aphorism "surgeons bury their mistakes" has more credence in the public view than might be anticipated. Absent some major quality effort by surgeons themselves, the federal government and insurance companies are likely to lay down the law, and demand changes in practice patterns which are based on uninformed data. The result will be a perverse reversal of what was actually intended.

What could happen on a large scale has already happened on a small scale. A decade ago Medicine began publishing unadjusted mortality rates for individual cardiovascular surgeons in western New York State. These were unadjusted rates, meaning that there was no risk adjustment calculation included. One surgeon could easily have had a practice consisting of urgent and emergent referrals of the worst kind, could have done a fine job with them, but looked bad in press. Moreover, the system in which the surgeon practiced was not considered. An operative result is more than the procedure itself, and involves the competency of anesthesia, postoperative recovery care, floor nursing, ancillary services, and many other factors. These considerations fell on deaf ears and the result was predictable. Surgeons began selecting the most straightforward cases, and referring difficult high-risk cases out of state. Society still had the problem patients, but they weren't in New York, and unadjusted mortality rates fell.

It's hard to view the federal government too harshly, since there was really no other good quality measurement available. The discipline of surgery had not provided one. For the same underlying reason, a group of very large and well-meaning employers, the Leapfrog Group, recently banded together and developed referral guidelines for their collective membership. This group holds considerable sway, being comprised of some of the world's largest corporations. The referral guidelines, rather than based on direct quality outcomes, were instead based on volume, thought to be an indirect proxy for quality. This is to say that for certain procedures (open heart, coronary catheterization, abdominal aortic resection, carotid endarterectomy, esophagectomy) a certain volume threshold must be met by a hospital before a Leapfrog Group member may undergo surgery at that hospital. This proxy is far from perfect, and on intense debate about the validity of the underlying assumption is ongoing. Again, it seems to be a question of nothing better being available.

Administrative databases (Medicare, HCFA) are frequently used to judge quality, but the data is unreliable. The University Hospital Consortium (UHC) is a prominent database that uses administrative data. Non-medical personnel paw through large stacks of charts and might be easily misled by complex medical situations. The data is retrospective, and frequently suffers from coding bias, in which an institution codes to maximize reimbursement rather than for accuracy. It is frequently impossible from a retrospective review to distinguish preoperative co-morbidities from true postoperative complications. Finally, a lack of standardized definitions from survey to survey invalidates the quality comparisons.

What any reliable quality indicator needs, and what the above mentioned do not have, is a solid risk adjustment methodology. Risk adjustment allows for comparisons of results between hospitals. Theoretically risk adjustment could be used to compare the results of individual surgeons, but usually one surgeon does not do enough of the same type of case to provide for statistically significant comparisons. Further, the patient risk adjustment does not account for deficiencies in systems, as was mentioned. Thus, risk adjustment is a process that is essential, but should be applied only to hospital populations for use in hospital-to-hospital comparisons. When variances are noted in hospital results in a particular specialty, then more focused interventions can be accomplished.

Surgeons in the past have been reluctant to expose their results because the methodology was flawed. The surgeons of the future must develop methodologies which will allow meaningful comparisons of hospital systems, with identification of best practices, and subsequent education in these areas. The focus on the individual should be minimized, except as egregious problems are discovered at a local level, by a chief-of-surgery or chief-of-staff. In this way, the surgeon of the 21st century, convinced that he is being judged fairly and objectively, and as part of a larger team, will be enthusiastic about sharing results, and learning from them. Society, likewise, should be satisfied that the surgical discipline is engaged in constructive self-evaluation.

There is a model of surgical outcomes reporting that fits the needs of both the discipline of surgery and society. In the future, this model will be a feature of every hospital providing surgical services. The National Surgical Quality Improvement Program, was conceived and incubated in the VA Health System and is now ready to be hatched into the private sector.(12-14) The important features of NSQIP are that it is prospective, it uses standardized definitions, utilizes a fixed endpoint (30-day mortality and morbidity), and nurse reviewers collect and enter data into a data collection system. Regular educational conferences are held for the nurse coordinators, and measures of interrater reliability are regularly obtained.

Most importantly, the NSQIP has developed a model for risk adjustment that works. Dozens of pieces of preoperative data are collected for each patient, using standardized rules, and entered into a predictive model which was derived from many thousands of patients. Using the model derived from the entire population of patients, and based on individual variables, an "expected" 30-day mortality and morbidity may be derived from each individual patient. When summed, these data are the "expected" mortality and morbidity for each individual hospital in the system, or for any subgroup. The actual 30-day mortality and morbidity is determined and results are presented as the observed/expected ratio (O/E ratio). In this way hospitals may be compared along a continuum of O/E ratios. The "our patients are sicker than yours" argument does not hold water in this system.

That risk adjustment changes one's perspective on the quality of surgical services is clear. The various arms of society interacting with the surgical disciplines need to appreciate this truth: unadjusted mortality rates are easy to collect but are misleading. This relationship is demonstrated below. Here hospitals are ranked in descending order of "quality" based on the unadjusted mortality rates, and then ranked according to O/E ratios. The crisscrossing pattern demonstrates how dramatically the ranking system changes with risk adjustment.

The most important aspect of this approach is that when quality hospitals are reliably identified, teams of informed surgeons can visit these hospitals, identify best practices, and distribute this information to hospitals of lesser quality. In this way the practice of surgery will make concrete advances on a regular basis.

In the future, surgery needs to adopt the NSQIP model or something similar to every hospital offering surgical services. Participation should be mandatory for accreditation. Data collection should be a part of the pre-hospital or in-hospital process. Intraoperative variables should be entered at the time of surgery, in the OR. Mortality models will be developed from the perspective variables alone, and before surgery the surgeon will have the predictive mortality and morbidity data to share with the patient, if he chooses.

It should be possible to apply the risk adjustment model to hospital cost data, and it may be possible to develop O/E ratios for hospital cost. In this way insurers will have access to the data they want, which will identify hospitals with good O/E ratios for survival, but also good O/E ratios for cost. Contracts may then be developed between hospital and insurance based on this data. Contracts may also be developed specifically for high risk patient populations, as defined by the universally accepted risk adjustment method. Results can then be compared from one tertiary care center to another for this level of care.

The anonymity of the results reporting is an issue under much discussion. Currently in the NSQIP, the results are anonymous, and this helps to insure participation. In the future, however, I doubt that results will remain anonymous. Hospitals will be ranked by O/E ratio in Newsweek, for all the public to see. This is not necessarily a bad evolutionary direction, however because with this data presentation will have to come some basic understanding by the public as to what quality really is. Anything will be better than the current ranking systems. It is really anybody's guess as to what goes into ranking the nation's best hospitals", but it is likely an amalgamation of "reputation", patient satisfaction and ease of parking.

The surgeon of the future must look within to re-calibrate the surgical life, and the discipline of surgery must look within to demonstrate to society what surgical quality really is. This may represent something of a sea change for us, but the future depends on it.

REFERENCES

1. Aufses AH, Slater GI, Hollier LH. The nature and fate of categorical surgical residents who "drop out". Am J Surg 1998;175:236-9.

2. Charlton J, Kelly S, Dunnel K, et al. Suicide deaths in England and Wales: Trends in factors associated with suicide deaths. Popul Trends 1993;69:34-42.

3. Vaillant GE, Sobowale NC, McArthur C. Some psychologic vulnerabilities of physicians. N Engl J Med 1972;287:372-5.

4. Murray RM. Psychiatric illness in male doctors and controls. An analysis of Scottish inpatient data. Br J Pscyhiatry 1977;13:1-10.

5. Green A, Duthrie HL, Young HL, PetersTJ. Stress in surgeons. Br J Surg 1990:77:1154-8.

6. Kobasa SC. Stressful life events, personality and health: an inquiry into hardiness. J. Pers Soc Psychol 1979;37:1-11.

7. Krizek TJ. Ethics and Philosophy Lecture: Surgery...Is it an impairing profession? J Am Coll Surg 2000;194:352-366.

8. Maslach C, Jackson S. Maslach Burnout Inventory. PaloAlto, CA: Consulitng Psychologists Press, 1986.

9. Campbell DA, Sonnad SS, Eckhauser FE, Campbell KK, Greenfield GL. Burnout among American Surgeons. Surgery 2001;130:696-705.

10. McCue JD, Sachs CL. A stress management workshop improves residents' coping skills. Arch Intern Med 1991;151:2273-77.

11. Mushin IC, Matteson MT, Lynch EC. Developing a resident assistance program. Arch Intern Med 1993;153:729-33.

12. Khuri SF, Daley J, Henderson W. Hur K, Gibbs JO, Barbour G, et al. Risk adjustment of the postoperataive mortality rate for the comparative assessment of the quality of surgical care: results of the national Veterans Affairs Surgical Risk Study. J Am Coll Surg 1997, 185(4):315-327.

13. Daley J., Khuri SF, Henderson W, Hur K, Gibbs JO, Barbour G, et al. Risk adjustment of the postoperative morbidity rate for the comparative assessment of the quality of surgical care: results of the National Veterans Affairs Surgical Risk Study. J Am Coll Surg 1997, 185:328-340.

14. Daley J, Forbes MG, Yung GJ, Charns MP, Gibbs JO, Hur K, et al. Validating risk-adjusted surgical outcomes: site visit assessment of process and structure. J Am Coll Surg 1997; 185:341-351.

CHAPTER 3

OPERATING ROOMS OF THE FUTURE

BRUCE C. STEFFES, M.D., LAZAR J. GREENFIELD, M.D.

The operating room has long maintained a mystique, a sense of holy sanctuary where surgeon-scientists practiced their ritual and art. The ancient concept of physician-priest was reinforced by the odd smells, blood and violation of the sanctity of the human body. As Berguer has written, "To maintain a strong commitment to the welfare of an individual patient, surgeons train and practice in such a manner that emphasizes the endurance of physical, mental and emotional strain. Such steadfast commitment to the patient, coupled with a very high socio-economic status, has understandably propelled most surgeons to see themselves as craftsmen-scientists (and perhaps as artists) and to be reluctant in allowing others to analyze their unique work environment".(1)

Ergonomics and work flow study of the operating room (OR) has been looked at sporadically, but no extensive study or wide-spread application of findings occurred. Operating rooms were looked at either as cost-centers (in governmental, institutional or managed-care settings) or positive margin-centers (in third-party reimbursement systems that were competitive and physician-driven). The latter viewpoint did not inspire a critical analysis of the operating room environment since decisions were made largely on the basis of return on investment.

Since an operating room is the most expensive service a hospital can provide, no longer can it be considered an independent fiefdom, but its design must be subject to good business, work-efficiency, cost-effective, and ergonomic principles. Operating room design and process must take into account all shareholders within an institution to assure optimal "buy-in" as well as provide the best possible design for the facility. Much time and effort are required to accomplish a critical analysis of every work process and prioritization of the goals to be achieved. The process and types of questions for the planning group have bene reported.(2,3)

Design Concepts

Integration will be the hallmark of future designs. This includes not only the integration of imaging techniques within the operating room, but also the massive revolution in information technology.(4) The operating suite will not have the luxury of being isolated from the rest of the hospital; indeed, good patient care will require integration of stored patient data, reference databases and the concurrent consultations. An example would be requesting a. radiologist to view real-time direct ultrasound output from the OR for joint interpretation with the surgeon. The pathologist will also be able to visualize a tumor in situ for better consultation on the results of a biopsy. The use of telemedicine for teaching and consultation will also increase once the legal and technical issues are resolved.

Design will reflect function. The need for more ergonomically correct design of tables and chairs has been increased by minimally invasive surgery, where the reduction in the degrees of freedom from seven to four has created a series of injuries due to prolonged attempts to perform procedures using suboptimal ergonomic principles.(5) Less obvious but equally important in overall function is room position within the suite, as well as position of doors, lights, and laminar flow systems. Planning this will be facilitated by rapidly developing virtual reality software programming that allows the design of the proposed OR by each user. This will evolve to its use not only for design but also for simulation.(6) At some point, operations will be able to be performed in true virtual reality which will allow surgeons to polish their skills, residents to practice the operation before attempting it on patients, and the objective assessment of a surgeon's skills for the purpose of credentialing. In addition, it will be possible to model the placement of various pieces of equipment to test the effects of the proposed design. Virtual reality will allow each person with a specific role in the OR to utilize the design and make suggestions. As a result, anesthesia staff, nurses, operating room and x-ray technicians, and others can contribute to the functionality of the design to suit their specific needs.

The design will take into account the role that the room must fulfill. There are significant differences in rooms designed for outpatient, multipurpose use and those designed for robotically controlled, image-integrated subspecialty procedures. The operating suite designed for a boutique hospital is different from that of a tertiary care academic center. To require that all rooms meet the same standards is illogical and not cost-effective. Therefore, once there is agreement on the minimal standards consistent with patient safety for all operating rooms, the design can be tailored for its intended use.

The design must allow maximal flexibility since the requirement for change is the only constant. As technology improves at an increasing rate, the design must have the flexibility to accommodate. One important way to control costs and facilitate the adoption of new technology is the development of industry standards. For optimal effect, this flexibility must be based on industry-wide agreement on standards for sizes of connections, sizes of conduits, types of connectors, and other structural and power requirements. Interchangeability for easy exchange of one modality for another would be highly desirable. Admittedly, this will be difficult to accomplish because many technology companies are relatively small and it is costly for them to change. There is also the understandable desire for proprietary design that maintains the connection with the purchaser. It is also possible for standards to stifle innovation, so this approach should be ongoing and industry-wide.

Having stated those general concepts, it is interesting to speculate on what types of systems might be used in future ORs. The following scenario is an attempt to predict the applications of future technology.

Jack stepped up to the scrub sink. Of course, it really wasn't a scrub sink, those were a thing of the past but he still thought about skin preparation that way. He thrust his arm into the preparation device. As the familiar tingle enveloped his arms, Jack glanced idly into the operating room. He watched as the anesthetist secured the endotracheal tube. It had of course been placed and positioned in another room along with all of the sensing devices. One wouldn't use valuable operating room time for such routine things. However, she wasn't satisfied with it once the patient was in the room and had re-secured it. A quick snap of the sensor yoke had reestablished all monitor and gas lines and the patient was ready. It had been a long time since he had seen an endotracheal tube used but then again, it had been a while since he had operated on an obstructed colon cancer. In fact, it had been a long time since he had operated on a colon at all. With the diagnostic capabilities of the last 10 years and the newer antibiotics and oncologic treatments, colon surgery was fast in danger of going the way of ulcer surgery. "These young kids coming out soon won't even know how to do that kind of surgery," he thought in derision but he kept his politically incorrect thoughts to himself. He watched through the window as the anesthetist's lips moved. He knew she was speaking to the computer and the blinking display was the only indication that the computer now had taken complete control of the patient. The biosensors would monitor micro capillary perfusion and a dozen chemistries including oxygen, carbon dioxide, radical formation and stress hormones. The machine was capable of instantaneous identification of trends and the algorithms would automatically adjust the anesthetic agents and treat any unsuspected life-threatening changes – not that those occurred very often anymore. All of the environmental factors were controlled by the computer as well as infusion fluid temperatures and bed temperature.

The timing light switched colors as the skin prep machine changed from a microbiocidal spray to the polymer spray that would coat his skin with an ultra thin layer effective for six hours. Not that anything took that long anymore. As he withdrew his arms, the film dried instantaneously. The door to the OR automatically opened by sliding into the wall and the room sensor hooked to the computer silently documented the time and the fact that the surgeon had entered the room. Each member of the staff and the patient himself wore a similar device.

Smiling, he greeted his surgical technician. Lost in his reverie, he had not seen him enter the room from the anteroom and uncover his fully set up table. There was always pressure to put more and more cases through this room. It had been 8 minutes since the last patient had rolled out and he knew the administrator would be unhappy with this delay. Jack slipped into his sterile gown and gloves. These gloves were amazing, he thought. Gossamer thin, they were almost puncture proof and yet felt like a second skin. He particularly enjoyed the advertisement that popped up in his web journal. It showed a man trying to stab through these with a scalpel and finally succeeding only with a sledgehammer and razor sharp nail. He had of course been vaccinated against all of the known viruses and bacteria, but his training from years ago still echoed in the recesses of his mind that one could not be too careful. He heard the other member of his team speak to the computer, double-checking to make sure that the computer had properly identified the surgeon and reconfirming the type of case. As she spoke, he interrupted her and made some minor changes. Instantaneously the display panel changed appearance again as the machines were automatically configured to his new preferences and he knew that the continuous recording had begun. There was a barely audible whir as the table changed its configuration to his preferred height. Later, at his command, the ambient lighting would dim to improve their visibility. Everyone was wearing a form of heads-up display so that they were all able to stay focused on the business at hand, even when they had to look away to attend to other matters. Alarms would immediately be visible in their field of vision if something was out of the ordinary. The computer had already done a precheck to confirm that every piece of equipment was working and had duly noted the otherwise unrecognized fact that the light source was reaching the number of hours of use that would justify replacement before it failed. The biomedical department was silently notified.

As the technician sprayed the skin and applied the drape, Jack stepped to the wall screen and instructed the computer to display the selected diagnostic images he had noted earlier on the ward. He then instructed the computer to connect him to his office receptionist whose visage filled the screen immediately. He told her of his change in plans and his expected arrival and cut the communication. The screen reverted to the view of the patient.

After determining that everything was to his satisfaction, he picked up the handheld laser and made the incision. This device was a far-cry from the previous lasers of his youth and in a way he didn't fully understand, it combined technologies so that it made a carefully regulated and completely dry incision. No more bleeding from the wound. Since the tumor mass was relatively large, he made a longer than usual incision —four centimeters seemed to mock him as a bit barbaric compared to his usual. After creating the other small incisions, he inserted the devices and attached the robotic arms. He missed the camaraderie of working with another colleague, but this was faster and more certain. The controls of his instruments felt like they were an extension of his hands. Indeed, in a way they were, for they had been custom made for his huge hands and took into account that he was left-handed. That was certainly different from before – he had hated feeling so awkward using instruments made for everyone or more accurately perhaps, for no one. Reaching for the dissector, a bloodless plane developed as he rapidly mobilized the mass. His robotic arm assistant followed his commands manipulating the lights and suction to keep his field of vision clear at all times. Suddenly frowning, he recognized a distortion in the anatomy near the great vessels that he had not appreciated before. Stepping away from the table, he asked the computer to isolate the course of the iliacs. A three-dimensional representation was immediately visible and he asked it to rotate back and forth. He then asked for an overlay of the tumor. Indeed, he had missed that subtlety before. Stepping back to the table, he spoke to the computer and a three-dimensional image suddenly appeared superimposed over his instruments and the tumor. As he twisted the tumor, the image stayed right with his movements. He was now easily able to isolate the blood supply to the tumor and dissect it off of the adherent vessels. He reflected back to the days of his residency when he would have done a more radical dissection. With the treatments available that was no longer necessary. The limited dissection was one of the many things that made post-operative ileus now a medical curiosity.

Now working with complete concentration, he sealed and divided the two ends of the colon. These new devices were based on ultrasonic vibration and could seal the protein of the wall, fusing the sides or an anastomosis into a strong bond. Done properly, leaks were a thing of the past. He carefully applied the tissue gel along the side of the anastomotic line and watched it change color rapidly curing into strong elastic tissue glue. Satisfied with his job, he instructed the camera to take a quick look around the abdomen. Given the new diagnostic imaging techniques, it was rare that anyone found something unexpected, but old habits died hard.

As the technician approximated the tissues, he applied the tissue gel to the fascial planes and finally to the skin. The technician would dress the wound with a biofilm after applying the electrodes that would keep the patient pain-free in the post-operative period. He still had things to do. Conscious of being somewhat of an anachronism, he still referred to it as "doing the paperwork." Stepping to the computer, he asked for a video connection to the waiting room and spoke to the family, reassuring them of the success of the operation. Next, he called up his standard orders. The computer noted his requested changes, double checked his orders against the pharmacy database and the patient's known drug and allergy profile and suggested a change. After approving the change, he then asked the computer to display the operative note. The computer had integrated the images he had selected during the case into the record. He dictated some changes which were made as he spoke. He read it quickly and "signed" it with his official voice print. As a matter of habit, he reviewed the entire documented record but as usual, it was textbook perfect. Out of curiosity, he called up the cost and time profile of this case, comparing it to both his previous profile and that of the average of his colleagues. Congratulating himself, he left the room wondering how he had ever tolerated the inefficiencies of the past.

Design for Structural Changes

Regardless of the technology that is developed, there will always be a need to transfer energy from the periphery of the room to a point near the patient. Whether that transfer of energy is done with hard-wiring (such as electricity, pressured gases, fiber optic cable) or whether it is can be done without hard-wiring (lasers, or electromagnetic radiation forms such as infra-red, radio, etc) will depend on future development.(7) The latter possibility will allow increased freedom of movement, less concern with cost of disposables and less concern with draping. Ceiling mounted arms will be used increasingly, both as a form of umbilical cord to get power and energy sources near the surgeon and to contain the technology which cannot, for various reasons, be removed from close proximity to the patient. The flexibility of the arm will allow variations in position of the arm and its connection points as well as the table and lights so that the room can be used for several types of procedures while retaining its usable space. The fact that the floor is clear makes movement around the room during an operation much safer and also facilitates cleaning between cases.

With proper design, such arms will have the long-term advantage of being re-wired easily to meet changing demands. It is likely that miniaturization will allow these arms to become increasingly more flexible. Current designers must reach an acceptable compromise between bulk (which affects torque forces and weight requirements for the ceiling support) versus improved ability to accommodate new technology of unknown size and wiring demands. Larger arms have more room for various cords, tubes and cables. Here again, industry wide standards will allow the arms to be mounted with a reasonable expectation that new pieces of equipment will fit and power lines and cords will be accommodated. When the room needs to be remodeled, it will then be a simple matter to place the device and technology suitable for that specialty into the existing ceiling arms.

There are some alternatives that bear consideration.(8) The first is a mobile terminus that sits on the floor but is connected by an umbilical cord to a locus on the wall. A clear advantage of such a system would be that it would be cheaper. The cord would have to be constructed to avoid kinking of gas or fiber optic lines and would have the obvious drawback of an obstacle on the floor. However, it would have the benefit of greater convenience of placement without need for extensive ceiling buttressing. This would be a good alternative for the lost-cost outpatient operating room. Another alternative is a floor terminus or one that came from the table itself. However, by definition this would tend to be fixed in one location or have a minimal range of movement, thereby limiting flexibility of table and light position. It would also be more difficult to service and to remodel the room unless the space beneath the floor was easily accessible. This is unlikely with the traditional poured concrete floor which would make this a less than desirable solution.

The last alternative is a floor that is easily adaptable. In the early days of large mainframe computers, flooring was developed that allowed the cables and cords to course beneath the floor. This would allow the terminus to be moved or be in multiple locations. Designed properly, a small terminus could be rolled into position over the desired point of connection and then "locked" into place for simultaneous connection of all lines at once. This system could have flexibility equal to ceiling mounted arms, but problems of resistance to water, strength of connections and ability to be cleaned easily would need to be addressed.

From an architectural standpoint, the shell of the operating rooms will need to have considerable flexibility. Ceilings must be high (a minimum of 10 feet) with sufficient bracing to handle considerable loads while providing room for the necessary tubing, plenums, laminar air flow systems and smoke evacuation systems. With the increasing rate of change in operating room requirements, modular construction or the use of non-weight bearing walls may have advantages. Such a design might result in a higher initial cost but would ultimately be cost effective over the course of 20 or 30 years from lower remodeling costs. It would also allow a faster remodeling process. Along with this flexibility, architects must appreciate the increased need for storage which has doubled or tripled with the advent of minimally invasive surgery.(9) Increased support space (for plenums, power, air-handling, etc) and for flexibility in electrical, water and drainage systems must be provided. When minimally invasive techniques were introduced, the space required for an average general surgical case increased about 50% and will undoubtedly increase further with the addition of robotics and integrated imaging systems. With careful design, it should be possible to have modular rooms that could be configured for certain types of cases and then reconfigured or replaced as necessary without months of disruption.

Carrying this concept to an operational level, the well designed OR should accommodate various specialties with minimal alteration. The design should allow rapid conversion between minimally invasive procedures and open cases and to allow easy conversion from the equipment needed for one specialty to that needed by another. There are several anesthesia systems which work on such a modular principle. For example, in surgery, to switch from a cholecystectomy case to knee arthroscopy, the insufflator cartridge could be exchanged for a cartilage shaver motor. With a standardized yoke, the carbon dioxide would automatically shut off and the electrical connection be established.

Equipment Considerations

Manufacturers should commit to standards within their own line of products that are designed with a ten to fifteen year life expectancy to warrant the major OR renovations necessary for installation. This combined with miniaturization will lower cost over the life of the equipment and is more ecologically sound, which will be increasingly important in the future. Ideally, equipment will be designed on a basic functional platform with the ability to add desired items from a menu. This will allow tailoring to both needs and budget. The design must also allow separation of the active modality and the controls. This minimizes the space requirements near the patient and allows one-point computer control and documentation.

Equipment design should also permit both front and back access with nurse-controlled access and controls placed on the side away from the sterile field. Duplicate gauges or indication lights would be mounted on the side toward the surgeon for monitoring or preferably displayed on the monitor. Ideally, compartments in the cabinet or shell of the ceiling arms would function as the outer case of each device to diminish weight and size. Such an approach would require standards for the size of the compartment which would allow subsequent innovations (e.g. 3-D screens, argon cautery, ultrasound, Doppler, cautery grounding systems) to be installed. The electronics for each type of unit would be mounted on removable (and updatable) cards for ease in maintenance and renovation. For example, failure of a power source would allow it to be removed and replaced with another unit kept in the operating room suite for just such an emergency.

As noted in the futuristic scenario, all devices and equipment would be in constant contact with and under the control of the computer.(10) It would automatically document their identification numbers, track usage hours for maintenance and regulate power levels and usage. Various surgeons' preferences would be set automatically by the computer.

One of the arguments against multiple specialty use of a room is the wide spectrum of supplies needed for different specialties and varied cases. One approach that would allow an adequate and accurate inventory is an improved cart system for quick conversions. When there was a need to convert from one specialty or one procedure to another, a tall wheeled cart behind a wall of glass doors would be wheeled out and a new one wheeled in and locked into place. These would be standardized for inventory and have a built-in bar-code reading device. They would be stocked in a central sterile area in another part of the hospital by trained technicians who would consult computerized lists of equipment. Nurses would not necessarily be involved, thereby saving costs. During a case, as supplies were used, they would automatically be passed over the bar-coding device. The computer would track actual utilization patterns by surgeon, specialty and case. This would become part of the computerized record for accurate charge generation and inventory control, not only for the cart but also for purchasing. When the cart was returned to the central sterile area, the technician would obtain a read-out of the supplies used and then replace them. This would minimize the operating room inventory of supplies but would likely increase the number of certain instruments needed. This more accurate mechanism of inventory control would prevent losses from uncharged items, prevent shrinkage from theft and facilitate a cost-effective just-in-time form of inventory management.

Instrument design will have undergone a major revolution since current instruments date back to the time when blacksmiths forged tools. The axes of the instruments should be in line with the axis of the forearm, hand and index finger.(11) It should also be feasible for the computer to scan a surgeon's hand and design an instrument specifically for that surgeon. This would be most valuable for needle-holders and other instruments used with great precision and less valuable for hemostats and other types of clamps. Therefore, someone with size 5 hands and left hand dominant would not have to use the same instruments that a right-handed, size 8.5 surgeon uses. Sterilization of instruments can also be improved. Treatment of instruments with various polymerization techniques and automation of equipment cleansing will improve both the cleaning process and create an anti-microbicidal film.

Instrument trays will be individualized and therefore have fewer instruments which will be pre-counted. Pre-counting requires that concomitant liability issues be addressed, perhaps by changing protocols or by reassigning registered nurses to the central sterile area. It is certainly more cost-effective to buy more instruments than to stop in the middle of the day to clean and resterilize equipment. Loss of income-producing OR time is a true opportunity cost and must be balanced against other expenses. It is not likely that disposable instruments will have replaced reusable ones.

Workflow and Documentation

The design of future ORs must reflect and enhance the intersecting work flows of various groups including nurses, anesthesia staff, surgeons, patients, sterile supplies, and the scrub team. The design process must begin from patient admission from the outpatient department and continue to discharge.(12) Since the highest efficiency of the OR is desirable, any process that is performed in that room that could reasonably be performed elsewhere is counterproductive to that goal. Just as it is beneficial for the anesthesia team to place an epidural and all invasive monitoring lines in another room while the operating room is in use, it seems appropriate for the scrub technician to set up the sterile table in an adjacent room in order for the prepared patient, the anesthesia team and the surgeon to arrive in the recently vacated and cleaned room at the same time. This is preferable to the staged approach that is wasteful of the resources of time and personnel.

Much time and effort is wasted in documenting by hand what can be documented electronically. A good example is the concept of computer based anesthesia records.(13) In the operating room of the future, not only will all the metrics (EKG, monitoring strips, EEG, gas flows, blood pressure) be recorded automatically, but advanced algorithms will allow the computer to monitor and predict physiologic responses so that gas flow and anesthetic agents can be adjusted automatically. Other metabolic states will be monitored including effects of co morbidities and current medications so that cardiac function and homeostasis are preserved. The entire environment of the operating room will be computer regulated so that ambient temperature, cooling and warming blanket temperature, temperature of intravenous fluids and airway humidity are monitored and adjusted to meet the needs of the patient.

As part of the computerized operating room, much of the documentation that consumes the nurse's time will have been automated. To use expensive personnel to document non-cognitive and non-interpretative events is counter-productive. The patient's armband will have a memory chip with a unique identifier and the computer will have documented the time of arrival and departure of the patient in the operating room as it will do within all areas of the hospital. Since the chip will have a complete medical history including past anesthetic complications, allergies, and current medications, the computer will be able to monitor the extensive database of drug interactions and modify its selection and administration of drugs accordingly.

With a completely computerized record of the clinical utilization patterns of time and resources, a valid cost analysis can be obtained. The surgeon will be able to compare his or her utilization pattern against the average to determine whether he is performing in a cost-effective way. This will assist the leadership of the institution in budgetary planning for equipment and supplies, investment in new programs and personnel, and justify rewards for improved quality of care parameters and behaviors that enhance effective utilization of the OR. More accurate information about utilization and efficiency will allow a better balance between the demands created by peak flow and unused time. Since turnover time can only be reduced so much, there is more to be gained by making the room more conveniently designed and ergonomically correct so that case length is more predictable and shorter.(14) This has the added benefit of a reduced patient complication rate since the incidence is known to be related to operative time. Accurate information about a surgeon's average case times and variability will also allow more rational scheduling.

Communications

During an operative procedure, the surgeon may have need for intermittent or continuous communication with imaging studies, laboratory data, past hospital records, the rest of the hospital, his or her office and occasionally home.(15) Using the same voice recognition or the sterile touch screen that is being used to control the robotic instrument holders and other operating room devices, it will be possible to bring up the scans and review them in real time with the radiologist, who can see both the images and the operative findings. Telephone, internet and telemedicine connections will be available for immediate contact with the resources, printed, image or consulting, that are needed to make the appropriate decision.

Perhaps the most fruitful area of development is the melding of diagnostic and therapeutic imaging techniques within the OR. Minimally invasive procedures will no longer require a monitor except for use by observers and the surgical team. Heads-up displays which allow three dimensional or true holographic representation of the field will be the standard and they will be capable of immediate audiovisual signaling of any abnormality in physiological or equipment function. Similar integration of radiographic and magnetic resonance images with robotically controlled stereotactic equipment will be available.(16) This will not be limited to the cranium but will also allow the superimposition of holograms and videographic images while operating in the chest and abdomen. The use of virtual reality and holographic or some other sort of three-dimensional stereotactic imaging will allow extraordinarily precise targeting of lesions which will be most valuable in solid organs (brain, spinal cord, liver). This will not only facilitate brain tumor ablation, but also for solid tumors elsewhere, imaging techniques combined with holographic projection will be able to warn the surgeon of the proximity of a large vessel or duct that has been distorted from its normal position. Placement of sensors using nanotechnology in key anatomical positions will also allow the monitoring of organ function to assess the physiological response to the operative resection. The integration of robotic techniques with motion-compensating software will allow more extensive coronary bypass grafting on the moving heart than is currently possible (17) as well as intrapulmonary procedures without sacrifice of ventilation.

It is interesting to speculate on the future role of robots in the operating room. The current concept as an extension of the surgeon's operative role neglects the potential of a robotic assistant or even as replacement of other personnel. Such an investment will not only be cost effective from the standpoint of indefatigability and work record but also the significant advantage of improved precision of action.

Conclusion

We are poised on the brink of a new and exciting revolution in the design of operating rooms as technology improves the sophistication of equipment and communications. The ability to integrate imaging techniques and information technology in real time during an operative procedure will provide the surgeon with remarkable resources to improve the precision of the operation and therefore clinical outcomes. Designing for improved workflow and flexibility of operating rooms will be an appropriate offset to the cost of new technology which can be further justified by the expected adoption of industry standards that will allow less costly equipment upgrades. Robotic enhancement of surgical technique will likely be followed by other roles for robots and nanotechnology yet unimagined.

REFERENCES

1. Berguer R. The application of ergonomics in the work environment of general surgeons, Rev Environ Health, 1997-Apr-June; 12(2)99-106

2. Steffes, B. "An Ambulatory Surgery Center and Laparoscopic Surgery – Lessons from Experience", Seminars in Laparoscopic Surgery. Seminars in Laparoscopic Surgery, 6:2, March 99

3. Steffes, Bruce, WS Eubanks, P Shadduck. "Concepts in Operating Room Design: Creation of a Room Dedicated to Minimally Invasive Surgery", Surgical Services Management, Volume 3, No 10 October 1997

4. Hajdukiewicz JR, Vicente KJ, Doyle DJ, Milgram P, Burns CM. Modeling a medical environment; an ontology for integrated medical informations design, Int J Med Inf, 2001 June; 62(1):79-99

5. Berguer R, Forkey DL, Smith WD. Ergonomic problems associated with laparoscopic surgery, Surg Endosc, 1999 May; 13(5): 466-8

6. Radermacher K, von Pichler KC, Erbse S, Boeckmann W, Rau G, Jakse G, Staudte HW. Using human factor analysis and VR simulation techniques for the optimization of the surgical worksystem, Stud Health Technol Inform. , 1996:29;532-41

7. Kavic MS. Robotics, technology and the future of surgery, JSLS, 2000: Oct-Dec; 4(4):277-9

8. Selman T. Engineering for the operating room of the year 2010, Health Estate Journal, 1999 Oct;53(8):18-20, 26.

9. Herron DM, Gagner M, Kenyon TL, Swanstrom LL. The minimally invasive surgical suite enters the 21st century, Surg Endosc, 2001 Apr; 15(4):415-22

10. Visarius H, Gong J, Scheer C, Haralamb S, Nolte LP. Man-machine interfaces in computer assisted surgery, Comput Aided Surg, 1997;2(2):102-7

11. Berguer R. Surgical technology and the ergonomics of laparoscopic instruments, Surg Endosc, 1998 May; 12(5):458-62

12. Brown D. Maximizing service delivery: one OR's experience, Leadersh Health Serv, 1994 Nov-Dec;3(6):20-4

13. Lanza V. Automatic record keeping in anesthesia -- a nine-year Italian experience, Int J Clin Monit Comput, 1996 Feb;13(1):35-43

14. Brown DL, Haward M. Key factors in improving surgical resources, Healthc Manage Forum, 1994 Fall;7(3):20-6

15. Gordon JL. Operating theatre information systems, Aust Health Rev, 1999:22(1):184-6

16. Heilbrun P. Image Guidance: the foundation for the future design of neurosurgical procedural facilities, Sterotac Funct Neurosurg, 1999;73(104);135-9

17. Boehm DH, Reichenspurner H, Detter C, Arnold M, Gulbins H, Meiser B, Reichart B. Clinical use of a computer-enhanced surgical robotic system for endoscopic coronary artery bypass grafting on the beating heart, Thorac Cardiovas Surg, 2000 Aug; 48(4):198-202

CHAPTER 4

ENVIRONMENTAL AND AESTHETIC CONSIDERATIONS

LAZAR J. GREENFIELD, M.D.

Traditionally, hospital and operating room planning were the province of experts with considerable experience whose focus was on efficient use of space and materials designed to satisfy physicians. Consultants were sought whose fundamental concepts often had originated under wartime conditions, so when the Trustees of Johns Hopkins estate were planning that hospital in 1874, they called on John Shaw Billings, whose experience was based on military hospitals (1), and the result was a pavilion-type facility that would support medical education. Today we recognize a broader commitment to satisfy the needs of many constituents including patients and their families, all healthcare providers, the community, varied payers and academic institutions and the government. Fundamental to successful planning is the realization that patients usually have a choice in selecting a hospital and that they no longer are willing to abdicate their autonomy nor sacrifice their comfort. For this reason, patients and community representatives must be involved in the planning process.

Patient and Family Concerns

Since patients associate quality of care with the quality of their hospital environment, it is important to understand their expectations. Patients and their families place high priority on good communication facilitated by easy connection to staff and caregivers. They value ease of access to an institution that is convenient and conducive to a sense of well-being. They expect respect for their privacy and confidentiality of their medical information in an environment that is safe and secure. They are also concerned about the risk of acquired infection and of operating room errors such as operating on the wrong side of the body. They value caring consideration of their family and of any impairment that they have. To the extent possible, they would like to be close to nature and the outside world. Attention to these concerns reduces stress for hospital staff as well and serves to reduce turnover.

Sources of stress for patients and families are not limited to anxiety about illness, its treatment, or pain, but also from confusion about directions, loss of control, lack of information or a non-caring attitude from staff or physicians. Much can be done to improve the entry process, and future hospitals will promote internet use for prior authorizations, registration, directions and parking. Although it is difficult to predict the nature of future medical payment plans, we can only hope that some form of single payer system evolves that will minimize the difficulties everyone endures with current insurance and health plans, geographical disparities in access and quality of care, and even attempting to understand professional and hospital bills. For hospital staff and physicians, stress comes from excess workload, problems with supervision and a frustrating work environment. Since the effects of these stressors are both psychological and behavioral, hospitals are well advised to utilize evidence-based design concepts to renovate as well as build new facilities. But what is evidence based design?

Evidence Based Hospital Design

There are five areas of research that have provided guidance for measurable improvements in the hospital environment. The first is in access to nature where indoor plants and gardens, outdoor gardens, nature views, both artificial and real, and natural light have been evaluated. (Fig. 1) Their use has been demonstrated to reduce

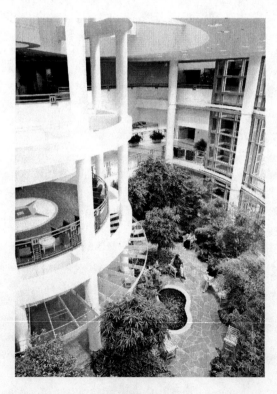

Figure 4-1
Incorporation of garden setting in the hospital. (Bronson Hospital, Kalamazoo, Mi, Larry Wolf, Photographer)

length of stay for psychiatric patients and to reduce stress for both patients and staff. The second is in control, where patients should be reminded that they have options and choices regarding their care and have access to privacy. Of equal importance is way finding which is facilitated by spacing of signs in hospital corridors every 150-200 feet and where more signs are placed at key decision points. The third area is the provision of positive distractions to include play areas for children, adding water to the nature areas and providing pleasant diversions such as art and music. One study by Menegazzi, Paris and Kersteen (2) showed that headset music provided to patients undergoing laceration repair was associated with less perceived pain. The fourth area is social support which includes cultural sensitivity and special provisions for family members. In addition, furniture that is arranged in group seating improves social interactions and has been demonstrated to lower seclusion rates and casualty incidents among patients with severe mental retardation. The fifth area is attention to environmental stressors such as noise, oppressive glare and light levels, and poor air quality. The physical danger of excessive light levels has been demonstrated in neonatal ICUs where premature infants exposed to brighter lights had a higher incidence of retinopathy.(3) There are additional advantages to retrofitting conventional light fixtures by installing energy-efficient electronic ballasts and T8 lamps, and replacing incandescent exit lights with LED technology including resource conservation and significant cost savings. The concept of building "green" hospitals that are resource efficient structures has gained wide support. This includes reduced energy and water consumption, improved indoor air quality, minimized impact on ecosystems and lowered hazardous waste production to obtain both cost and societal benefits. In addition, government agencies are issuing mandates for sustainable design and have adopted the Leadership in Energy and Environmental Design (LEED) rating system developed by the U.S. Green Building Council to evaluate a building's environmental performance over its life cycle.(4) The General Services Administration now requires that all federal capital projects beginning in 2003 meet the minimum requirements for LEED certification which includes site sustainability, water efficiency, energy and resource use, indoor environmental quality, and innovation and design processes. As an added incentive, government agencies now link tax credits to the adoption of green building practices.

Hospital and operating room requirements will differ depending on whether or not the facility has an obligation for teaching and training. Educational needs include space for teaching, parking, call rooms and lockers as well as access to information resources including computer work stations and a library. The rapid proliferation of image-based diagnostic and therapeutic procedures has amplified the need for easier physician and trainee access to images. In this situation, the traditional film-based approaches in radiology can not scale sufficiently to keep pace. As a result, many institutions have invested in new technology for Picture Archiving and Communication Systems (PACS). This approach archives digital images from a variety of imaging sources such as standard x-ray, CT and MRI scans and ultrasound, and allows them to be viewed at multiple locations electronically. Although such an investment in PACS is expensive, there is evidence of both increased operational efficiency and cost savings when compared to the cost of traditional production and storage of images. Future developments in technology will undoubtedly simplify this process and reduce the costs. However, such technology includes the downside risk of system failure obligating the institution to have plans for disaster recovery and backup to minimize data loss and service disruption.

The Center for Health Design (CHD) is a nonprofit, non-membership research and advocacy organization established in 1988 to promote the visionary idea that the design of the built environment can enhance the quality of healthcare. Over the first decade of its existence, it was able to educate healthcare and design professionals at its annual Symposium on Healthcare Design, to fund research on consumer satisfaction, medical outcomes and facility design, and to advocate new standards for the Joint Commission on the Accreditation of Healthcare Organizations. Now in its second decade, it has added the concept of partnerships with selected innovative healthcare organizations for specific projects to serve as examples that can be shared with other institutions throughout the world. This has been named the "Pebble Project" to simulate the effect of tossing a pebble into a pond. The desired ripple effect in the healthcare community will come from the documented results of projects that have created what are called life-enhancing environments for patients, families and staff.

The prototype Pebble Project was created in 1999 as a partnership between San Diego Children's Hospital, Anshen and Allen Architects and CHD. The result is a $25 million Children's Convalescent Hospital that will open in 2002. The project has studied how organizational behavior changes as a result of the planning and design process and will use standardized evaluation methodology for comparison of outcomes, identification of best practices and continuous improvements of healthcare design. It is expected that other projects will measure patient, family and staff satisfaction in both old and new facilities and use the data to gauge the cost-effectiveness of the approach.

Other partnerships involving adult hospital facilities have featured design changes to minimize patient transfers such as combining ICU and step-down units, placing flat-panel computers outside each patient's room for patient data handling which also allows patient and family use for e-mail, internet or games, and constructing parking that is aligned horizontally with each level of the hospital.(Fig. 2) (5) Some hospitals have taken the next step of offering resort-style amenities to attract patients such as fine food, golf-cart shuttles, satellite television, pay-per-view movies, individualized musical therapy and terrycloth robes. These amenities are used in the most competi-

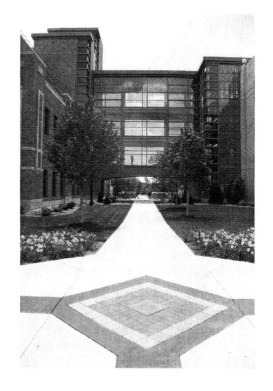

Figure 4-2
Alignment of hospital visitor parking with each level of the hospital (Bronson Hospital, Kalamazoo, Mi, Larry Wolf, Photographer)

tive markets and for selected populations such as obstetrics. In the future, it seems likely that hospitals will use marketing data to design their facilities and will target specific areas such as cardiovascular, orthopedic or ophthalmologic disorders that allow for more customization of facilities. There are, in fact, examples of extending this concept to hospitals including "surgical hospitals" which bridge the gap between ambulatory surgery centers (ASCs) and general hospitals. Incentives for this include enhanced reimbursement, physician interest and consumerism favoring specialty centers of excellence. Enhanced reimbursement results from the ability to bill for procedures not otherwise allowed under the restrictions on ASCs by Medicare and other payers. Physicians are attracted by dedicated services, absence of emergency or complex cases which alter operative schedules and lower rates of infection. Although ASCs can utilize an extended recovery care designation, the unlimited length of stay of a surgical hospital is much preferred by patients to the 23 hour limit of the extended care ASC. Patients also enjoy the atmosphere of a smaller facility with easier parking, nature areas and other amenities such as a drive-through pharmacy. We can expect to see more experimentation with this concept according to the newly formed American Surgical Hospital Association. Hospitals will have to choose their investments carefully balancing cost-effectiveness with the need to remain competitive.

Operating Room Considerations

Like the hospital environment, the patient's perception of quality of care in the operating room is based to a large extent on the projected image of the facility. This will include its visual appeal, convenience, comfort, speed of processing and friendly, professional image. Decisions regarding location and site of the facility will depend on whether one is dealing with inpatients or exclusively with outpatients in a dedicated ASC. The latter is perhaps the easiest to define since the prime consideration is ease of access for patients via major thoroughfares and adequate space for parking. Some proximity to a hospital is necessary, however, for the unexpected events that require patient transfer and hospitalization. For the community that will house the ASC, there will be legitimate concerns regarding its impact on traffic flow, and for its requirements for power, water and sewer connections. Security may also be a consideration if any abortions are performed in the facility or if it is intended for use by incarcerated patients. On a positive note, there are economic benefits for the community in terms of job creation and the increase in business for motels or hotels in the area and for food service providers. Planners are well advised to spend time with local officials before any major investments are made in real estate or architectural services. For both ASCs and hospital ORs, planners must assume that the facility will succeed and that sufficient growth in workload will occur to require expansion or extended hours operation. Therefore, generous storage and workroom space should be included that would lend itself to future renovation or conversion to operating rooms.

Although the current economic environment for hospitals is particularly challenging with declining reimbursement, forced indigent care and escalating expenses, the operating rooms provide the highest margin for the institution and remain its best investment. That investment, however, must be designed for optimal productivity and efficiency delivered with a positive attitude by all involved personnel. Future requirements for more sophisticated equipment and technology dictate requirements for larger ORs that have multiple conduit access, larger workrooms for technical support and larger storage areas. These demands are easier to satisfy at locations away from major hospital centers where space and construction costs command a high premium. Therefore, we are likely to see a satellite system develop based on a "control center" that allows surgeons to operate through digital imaging and robotics on patients in ASCs that are more convenient and accessible. As discussed previously, more ASCs are likely to be specialized for a specific patient population that may be geriatric, pediatric, international, gender-specific, specialty-oriented, or ranging from welfare to luxury environment. Of course, hospitals will retain their need for ORs for the most complex and labor-intensive cases as well as to support their trauma and emergency services.

Inpatient ORs are less likely to be able to match the hotel image sought for the rest of the hospital, but family waiting areas will benefit from the amenities mentioned previously. In addition, private consultation rooms for discussions with the surgeon are important and should be equipped with display boards that the surgeon can use to illustrate what was done for the patient. Ready access for the family to play areas for children, reading material and television, food and beverages, telephones and clergy must be available. Positive distractions are helpful to families under these stressful circumstances and may include art, aquariums, headset music, and gardens or nature areas.

Design of the OR facility must consider traffic flow as well as spaces and systems. Good flow is the vascular system of the facility and must include considerations of distribution and interface of patients, medical and paramedical staff, equipment, sterile and nonsterile instruments and supplies, regular and hazardous refuse, pharmaceuticals, pathology specimens and radiographs, and biomedical engineering. The spaces and systems must be flexible and capable of responding to change with minimal disruption. Infection control and minimizing the risk of cross-contamination are of constant concern and can be addressed in facility planning by providing dedicated toilet facilities for patients, staff and visitors with adequate hand washing stations in both bathroom and nourishment areas. New American Institute of Architects (AIA) guidelines require that surgical suites have sufficient proximity storage to keep hallways free of equipment and supplies.(6) The guidelines define the requirements for maintaining a measurable air pressure differential in the OR that will require that the room be virtually airtight. This includes sealing of all wall penetrations, especially above ceilings. The ceilings must be non-textured and "monolithic" to facilitate aggressive cleaning. There are even new standards for the temperature of hot water requiring 105°F to 120°F expecting the higher temperatures to reduce the growth of Legionella. If a problem with that pathogen is identified, then the recommendation is to go even higher to 140°F which raises the risk of scalding. It seems likely that future methods of infection control will include better methods of both water purification and OR cleaning with the possibility that washing and vacuum cleaning will be built into OR walls and floors to automate the turnover process and further reduce OR personnel needs. Since staff salaries represent an estimated 80% of the cost of the area, this offers the greatest opportunity for cost savings. By centralizing functions and command points, more effective patient and facility management can be achieved. Design improvements can include nurse and bed station pods, shared preoperative and stage II recovery cubicles, centralized nurse work and administration, and electronic information transfer for medical records and supplies. Future surgical suites will automate most instrument and equipment needs for individual procedures and surgeons and it is likely that robotic development will allow that modality to serve as surgical assistants as well as extension of the surgeon's skill. Other developments in the field of nanotechnology will undoubtedly have applicability in both anesthesia and surgical management.

Conclusions

Increasing sophistication and expectations of patients and families make hospital and OR construction more complex and expensive at a time when payers are reducing reimbursement. The challenge is to meet the expectations in a cost-effective approach using evidence-based design concepts. Both new and unimagined future technological advances will be necessary to reach these goals and improve patient outcomes.

REFERENCES

1. Cameron JL. Early contributions to the Johns Hopkins Hospital by the "other" surgeon: John Shaw Billings. Ann Surg 2001; 234:267-278

2. Menegazzi JJ, Paris PM, Kersteen CH, Flynn B, Trautman DE. A randomized, controlled trial of the use of music during laceration repair. Ann Emerg Med 1991; 20(4):348-350

3. Glass P, Avery GB, Subramanian KN, Keys MP, Sostek AM, Friendly DS. Effect of bright light in the hospital nursery on the incidence of retinopathy of prematurity. New Engl J Med 1985; 313(7):401-404

4. Building construction: being "Green" is easier and more cost effective than it seems. Health Care Advisory Board-Cost and Finance Watch 2001; Vol 2, #42

5. Voelker R. "Pebbles" case ripples in health care design. J Amer Med Associa 2001; 286(14):1701-1702

6. Cowan T. The new AIA guidelines: their impact on pre and postop infection control. Infection Control Today 2001; Oct:40-42

CHAPTER 5

ROBOTICS IN SURGERY

JUAN ARENAS, M.D.

Introduction

Webster defines a robot as *"a machine that resembles a human and does mechanical, routine tasks on command."*

From his earliest beginnings, man understood the concepts of labor saving devices, and as time progressed, developed methods for making work easier via beasts of burden, inclined planes, wheels, pulleys, hydraulics, engines, and computers.

In many instances, literature preceded reality; for example, Dr Frankenstein's modern Prometheus by Mary Shelley written in 1818, or *Rossum's Universal Robots*, a play by Karel Capek written in 1920, in which Capek based the idea of a mechanical man or woman on the Czech word *robata* which meant drudgery or forced labor. In the play, set on a remote island in the mid-twentieth century, robots acquired human emotions, learned to resent their servility, and destroyed their masters. In 1941, Isaac Asimov adopted the term *robotic*, which he applied to methodology in industrial automation.(1) In 1968, Asimov described 3 laws of robotics:

1) A robot may not injure a human being, or, through inaction, allow a human being to come to harm.
2) A robot must obey the orders given to it by a human being, except when such orders would conflict with the first law.
3) A robot must protect its own existence, except where such protection would conflict with the first or second law.

For much of the last half of the 20th century, robots and robotics were key factors in both the industrial world and the realm of science fiction. Laparoscopy and the paradigm of minimally invasive surgery provided the entrée for robotics into contemporary surgical practice.

However, the terminology is not a perfect fit. *Rossum's Robots* and assembly-line robotics are, in a sense, independent automated contractors. They have been given a set of instructions (the computerized algorithm) and are then left relatively free of their human masters to do their jobs. Surgical robotics differs in that they are direct extensions of human thought and handwork. However, the robotic aspect allows for improved manual dexterity (e.g. no tremor), greater magnification, off-site surgical direction, and simultaneous real time observation and consultation by parties throughout the world.

The curiosity of surgeons in concert with market forces will continue to prompt and stimulate innovative changes. Solutions to many surgical problems will be continually forthcoming through advancements in robotic methodology. For other surgical problems, advantage will not accompany novelty.

Furthermore, the constraints of declining reimbursement will demand that substantial economic advantage in the health care system will be necessary to balance the huge costs of technology. The next generation of both surgeons and accompanying surgical facilities will need to be familiar with and friendly to 21st century surgical practice.

Background

We are only beginning to experience what were heretofore unimaginable technological innovations in surgical techniques. For the first time it is now possible for surgeons to perform surgery without direct visualization or physical contact with tissue. Minimally invasive surgery has not only altered the performance of specific operations but has also changed the algorithmic steps of many operative procedures. The pain, discomfort, disability, and other morbidities associated with surgery are typically related to the trauma involved in directly accessing an operative site. The concept of performing surgery through an endoscope dates to the late 19th century; however it was the technology of the 20th century that made endoscopic surgery commonplace. The following technological advances facilitated this shift:

(a) Development of the charged coupling device (CCD) chip that allows high resolution video images to be transmitted through an optical scope to the surgeon;

(b) High intensity xenon and halogen light sources that improve vision of the surgical field; and

(c) Innovative hand instrumentation for endoscopic approaches.(2)

Surgical procedures may be categorized in terms of complexity, namely excisional, whereby a structure is removed (appendix, gallbladder); ablative, whereby tissue is destroyed (cryosurgery, radio ablation); reconstructive, whereby structures are joined or connected (e.g. bowel or Fallopian tubes); or salvage procedures, whereby organs are removed intact and preserved for further use (e.g. living donor nephrectomy). By the early 1990's minimally invasive surgery became routine, allowing surgeons to perform many general endoscopic and orthopedic procedures by accessing surgical fields through small incisions, thereby eliciting less pain and shorter periods of recovery. However, several characteristics inherent to laparoscopic surgery have hindered its progress and diffusion into the surgical mainstream. These characteristics include:

The requirement for highly trained personnel to maintain instruments and assist during operative procedures, expensive disposable instrumentation, laparoscopic instruments of poor ergonomic design, two dimensional video presentation of a three dimensional operative field, working environments not conducive to operator comfort (e.g. poor monitor placement), limited ability to steer rigid instruments, and lack of haptic (touch) sense. Intense efforts are currently being made to alleviate these handicaps.(4)

We are presently on the threshold of the next phase in minimally invasive surgery, i.e., the use of robotics in surgery. This technology was developed in the automotive and defense industry, where it has improved accuracy and safety. Robotics have significantly changed and improved the production of cars, for example in Germany, 80% of the production of the new Audi 2 is performed by robots.(5)

Several surgical robotic systems have been introduced in Europe, including the AESOP and ARTEMIS. In the United States in July of 2000, the FDA approved Intuitive Surgical's DaVinci system; i.e. the application of robotic surgery, operating at a site remote from the surgeon. Transposition of surgical and technical expertise from one site to another (e.g. battlefield, space station, or developing country) was expected to expand surgical resources. The medical industry has utilized robots for automatic laboratory sampling, aids for handicapped patients, and devices for different surgical procedures.

The initial use of Robotics for improving instrument function was in endoscopic guidance, whereby robotic instrument holders were employed to direct the endoscope during surgery. These robotic manipulators proved to be safe and efficient and are now accepted as assisting devices among endoscopic surgeons.(6)

Robotic system technologies significantly impact work procedures in the operating room. The integration of the different devices used for endoscopic operations into system structures which are easy to control and to maintain, is an important prerequisite for optimizing and allocating surgical resources. Telecommunication technology applied to surgery will help leverage surgical expertise among centers, and facilitate information transfer and accelerate the diffusion of surgical techniques among leading centers.

Robotics in the "OR"

Minimally invasive interventions require a multitude of technical devices, such as cameras, light sources, and insufflations. The devices used today are typically stand-alone units that need to be moved to an operating room well in advance of procedures.

Cables and hoses connected from each of these individual devices can be quite lengthy and hazardous. A hodgepodge collection of devices, connectors, and personnel infringe on the sterility and available space in the OR. The human arm and hand, although marvelously bioengineered for specific tasks, are not adapted well to laparoscopic surgery. The arm-hand unit has seven degrees of freedom (DOF) that allow the hand precise manipulation in three-dimensional space. However, during minimally invasive surgery, the cannula diameter forbids ingress of the hand into the operative field, and is substituted by laparoscopic instruments. First-generation laparoscopic instruments proved to be poor substitutes for the hand and are limited in range to 4 degrees of freedom; the first 2 degrees of freedom concern rotation of the laparoscopic instrument around the point of insertion (I) and the X and Y planes. The third degree of freedom involves rotation around the shaft axis of the instrument. The fourth degree of freedom is a translation (in and out) movement of the instrument. Despite advances in instrument design, standard laparoscopic instruments at the beginning of the 21st century continue to permit only 4 degrees of freedom.(5)

A dramatic transition from the industrial age to the information age is currently underway. It is therefore plausible to suppose that the solutions for the current problems of minimally invasive surgery lie within information technologies. Much of what the physician does on a daily basis involves information management. Therefore, information technology and information equivalents may be used to resolve some of the hindrances currently inherent with minimally invasive surgery.

Robotics Today

Several devices replacing the camera operator are available to secure and manipulate laparoscopes:

(1) AESOP (Automated Endoscope System for Optional Positioning) can recognize voice commands. The system facilitates a laparoscopic procedure by abolishing the need for an assistant, providing stability of view, offers minimal inadvertent lens smearing, and results in less fatigue of the operative team. Visualization of the operative field remains under direct control of the surgeon, thus reducing the amount of personnel necessary for the procedure.

(2) HERMES is another device that enhances laparoscopic surgery. This voice-activated system recognizes spoken commands that can adjust lighting in the operating room, adjust the operating table, contact another physician, or gather information on the Internet. A wealth of information and databases can be therefore made available to the surgeon during a procedure.

---

1 AESOP arm (Computer Motion, Goleta, CA)
2 HERMES System (Computer Motion, Goleta, CA)

(3) ARTEMIS (Advanced Robotic Telemanipulator for Minimally Invasive Surgery) manipulator system has two basic components, the user station (master) and the instrument station (slave). The steerable instrument and guiding arm permit spatial mobility of the instrument tip with 6 degrees of motion freedom.

Scaling, which is a specific control feature of advanced manipulator systems, allows alteration of the ratio between the input and output movement of the system. This capability to scale movement, either upward or downward, results in more precision control by the surgeon during the procedure. Obviously this technology complements and enhances human performance.

(4) ZEUS is one such a remote-controlled robotic device. This device incorporates 3 remote controlled-interactive arms: one voice–activated arm to control the laparoscope, utilizing AESOP's technology, and 2 robotic arms to manipulate the desired instruments. Instruments at the end of the robotic arms are controlled with a joystick at the surgeon's workstation. Built-in tremor control dampens the natural tremor present in the human hand and allows for greater control of surgical instruments.

(5) DA VINCI surgical system combines robotics and computer imaging thus enabling microsurgery in a laparoscopic environment. The system consists of the surgeon's viewing and control console (workstation) integrated with a high performance, 3-dimensional monitor system, a patient bedside cart consisting of three robotic arms that position and maneuver the endoscope, endoscopic instruments and a variety of articulating instruments. The surgeon's hand, wrist, and finger movements are translated into corresponding micro-movements within the patient's body. Haptics are employed to reproduce the surgeon's hand movements in a restricted and confined space. The ability to perform precision manipulation endoscopically enables coronary artery bypass procedures on a beating heart, radical prostatectomy, and donor nephrectomy for kidney transplantation.

The Future

Surgery has a bright and promising future as it enters the 21st century. Robots are here to stay. By utilizing information technologies, cost savings will be realized by the decrease in the number of skilled assistants necessary in the OR, and the availability of more accurate and less traumatic operative procedures.

---

3 ARTEMIS (Karlsruhe Research Center, Karlsruhe, Germany)
4 ZEUS system (Computer Motion, Goleta, CA)
5 DA VINCI (Intuitive Surgical, Inc., Mountain View, CA)

Needless to say, thorough and adequate training and proficiency in traditional endoscopic techniques are prerequisites for robotic expertise. In the event that complications arise during a minimally invasive procedure, the surgeon must be prepared to quickly intervene with traditional open-surgical methodology. Surgical workstations remove surgeons from operative fields, thus reducing operator fatigue by improving ergonomics. Additionally, the operating team will be better protected from contagious or communicable disease. Eventually, with a surgeon trained in traditional open surgery standing by the patient, robotic techniques will allow specialists to perform complex operations at sites far distant from the patient (telesurgery). This will undoubtedly prove beneficial for patients in remote areas with otherwise no access to first-line technology.

Robotic surgery, when combined with other advanced computer-based technologies such as the three-dimensional CT scan, may permit preoperative modeling of the surgical field using sophisticated imaging techniques. Realistic simulation of the surgical area will serve to more precisely plan operations before they are actually performed. Complex operations such as liver and pancreatic resection may be performed robotically with greater ease and less risk. Customized software helps program robots to imitate a surgeon's movements, particularly in complex task performance such as knot tying. A Robot can be programmed to perform without the direct intervention of the surgeon.

To facilitate surgical training, new advances in surgical simulation by virtual reality technology have enabled the recreation of 3-dimensional images and models.

Despite the levels of sophistication achieved by high-resolution images, robotic operators are still unable to feel or touch tissue. Force (haptic) feedback instruments promise to fill that gap by adding sense of "touch" to the simulated world. Developed for telepresence laparoscopy, haptic devices (from the Greek haptesthai, meaning "to grasp or touch") facilitate the interaction between the robotic device and the surgeon.

Currently, one of the most sophisticated haptic feedback devices is known as the PHANToM (SensAble Technologies Inc, Woburn, MA). This interface interacts with a computer-generated virtual world, providing pitch, yaw and thrust capabilities. The PHANToM is well suited as a research tool in that it recreates the haptic sensation of a laparoscopic instrument operated in a virtual reality world or during telepresence surgery. NASA has developed what is known as the Sensor or Data Glove. This interface is wired with multiple sensors that translate the movements of the surgeon's hand to a robotic arm via a powerful processor. This wearable piece of hardware was first introduced in 1995, at which time its main function was to translate touch from a robotic arm onto the skin of the user.

An additional development in minimally invasive surgery instrumentation is MEMS (Micro Electro Mechanical Systems), a technology that integrates electronics with mechanical structures as small as millimeters to microns. MEMS technology may be applied to the development of a new generation of laparoscopic instruments with miniature grips that mimic the human hand, therefore providing more degrees of freedom. This instrument is assembled in a vertebrae configuration and integrated with silicon microsensors capable of differentiating thermal, or color changes, thus allowing the robot to process the information acquired by the sensors and respond appropriately.

The concept and development of blending instrument and energy sources as an aid to dissection will continue. Unfortunately the design and engineering of laparoscopic instruments frequently occurs in an environment other than the surgical arena. As a result, instruments may boast an array of clever new features from an engineering standpoint, however surgeons may find it to have poor performance and limited functionality for surgical purposes. It has become increasingly apparent that surgeons must be consulted in the early developmental phases of new devices and instruments.

One particular issue that must be considered very carefully with the introduction of this exciting technology is cost. Initial investment and operating costs for a robotic surgical device amount to approximately US\$800,000 and another US\$100,000 for annual maintenance. This engenders an approximate increase in cost per case of approximately US\$2000. Considering current reimbursement schedules, it is evident that few centers can afford such expenditure. In the future, collaboration between health care facilities and industry are absolutely necessary. Another major challenge will be to convince payors that the increased costs associated with such technology, using robotic systems, justify the investment. The biomedical research community must understand that the advancements that most likely will bring medical science to the next level, are not going to be exclusively at the biochemical and molecular level, but instead are going to involve biomechanics, new technology and new techniques.

This recognition is in concert with the expanded view of scholarship in medicine. Medical science will advance through the scholarship of discovery, the scholarship of integration, the scholarship of application, and the scholarship of education. A tour of these and similar areas of learning will advance the art and science of our surgical craft as it continues to become more minimally invasive.

REFERENCES

1. Marescaux J, Smith MK, Folscher D, Jamali F, et al. Telerobotic Laparoscopic Cholecystectomy: Initial Clinical Experience with 25 patients. Annals of Surgery Vol 234, No 1, 1-7, 2001

2. Chitwood WR, Nifong LW, Chapman WH et al. Robotic Surgical training in an Academic Institution, Annals of Surgery Vol 234, No 4 October 2001

3. Rassweiler J, Binder J, Frede T. Robotic and Telesurgery: wil they change our future? Current Opinion in Urology 2001, 11:309-320

4. Schurr MO, Srezzo A, Buess GF. Robotics and systems technology for advanced endoscopic procedures: experiences in general surgery. European journal of Cardiothoracic Surgery 16 9Suppl.2) (1999) S97-S105

5. Mack MJ. Minimally Invasive and Robotic Surgery JAMA, February 7, 2001- Vol 285, No 5

6. Park AE, Mastrangelo MJ, Gandsas A, et al. Laparoscopic Dissecting Instruments, Seminars in Laparoscopic Surgery, Volume 8, No 1(March), 2001: pp 42-52

CHAPTER 6

ANESTHESIOLOGY

KEVIN K. TREMPER, M.D., PH.D., JENNY J. MACE

Anesthesiology and the operating room have developed to compliment the advances in Surgery over the last century and a half. To gain an appreciation for these developments and what may come in the next century, let us look at the evolution of the operating room through the eyes of physicians born in the mid 19th, 20th and 21st centuries. The dramatic advances made in one lifetime make one prediction inevitable; the operating room will be a completely different place 100 years from today.

1850 to 1900

In the early 1800s a surgical procedure was a gruesome event. Most patients would approach it as they would an execution for the ultimate results may be similar. Their personal affairs would have to be put in order for if the shock associated with the procedure did not kill them, the postoperative infection most likely would. The patients were brought to the operating theater where their extremities were bound and in some cases the patients were hooded execution style so they would not be forced to view the event. In Boston, on October 16, 1846, an event occurred which was to change the course of surgery forever. WTG Morton, a practicing dentist and a second year medical student at Harvard, demonstrated the effects of inhaled ether in producing a state later named "anesthesia".(1) The surgeon was John Collins Warren, a Dean of Harvard Medical School, one of the founders of the Massachusetts General Hospital, as well as one of the original editors of the Boston Medical and Surgical Journal (which was to become the New England Journal of Medicine). 1 Another Harvard faculty, Oliver Wendell Holmes, was the individual who named this state of suspended animation as "anesthesia." Seven years later in England, John Snow used inhaled chloroform to reduce the pain of labor for Queen Victoria at the birth of Prince Leopold.(1) Over the next 25 years, the use of inhaled ether and chloroform became more common, although there were religious debates over the ethics of inducing such a state. Surgical procedures were also somewhat limited to superficial excisions and amputations because of the attendant postoperative infections of more extensive procedures.

In 1875 a young physician completed his one-year surgical training at the first teaching hospital in the United States, the University of Michigan Hospital (opened in 1869). As with all surgical residents at that time he was required to write a thesis.

His thesis was entitled "Anesthetics and Their Uses" and his name was R.H. Tremper.(2) It begins by stating that anesthesia "certainly deserves to rank as the most important improvement in modern medicine or surgery." In his 47-page treatise he reviews the discovery of the current anesthetics along with how they are chemically derived. He describes in detail their use along with the five stages or degrees of anesthesia. The fifth degree was described as "a state of impended respiration observed previous to death in animals killed by chloroform." The fourth degree was the state of "absolute relaxation of voluntary muscles." He also describes five principles that should be closely attended: recumbency, an empty state of the stomach, a free-play of the diaphragm, an abundance of atmospheric air, and gradual administration [of the anesthetic].(2) He emphasizes the importance of having an empty stomach "because if chloroform is given soon after a hearty meal it will be almost certain to induce vomiting." He also cautions that although the patients should not eat prior to the anesthetic, "the interval should not be too protracted less serious exhaustion will result." Henry Tremper also recommended the importance of careful titration of the anesthetic, of constant monitoring the respiration, and to feel the pulse of the patient. His thesis in 1875 encompasses many of the basic principles used in anesthetic practice today.

At the turn of the century, the operating room was still a theater and anesthetic equipment was limited to simple devices to produce vapors of ether and chloroform. During the same period Harvey Cushing (the renowned neurosurgeon) made several important advances in anesthesia which he practiced as a resident. He, along with Codman, developed the first anesthesia record in 1895 and was the first to measure blood pressure during anesthesia with a technique he learned from Riva-Ricci during a trip to Italy. 1 Cushing was later the first to appoint a physician to be head of anesthesia in an effort to improve training and safety.(1)

Twenty-five years after Henry Tremper's graduation from surgical training at Michigan, there were still no Anesthesiology journals, no societies and no training programs. It was not until 1936 that the American Society of Anesthesiologists was formed as an offshoot of the New York Society of Anesthesiologists. It had 484 members.

1950 to 2000

On January 5, 1948 Kevin K. Tremper was born. Another Tremper ultimately to develop an interest in anesthesiology. Several major changes had taken place since the previous Tremper wrote his thesis: antibiotics were available, sterile techniques were used in operating rooms and anesthesia machines were available which allowed anesthetic vapors to be given in relatively precise concentrations and mixed with a combination of oxygen and nitrous oxide. Carbon Dioxide (CO_2) absorbers were incorporated into these anesthesia machines so that the circle ventilation system could be used for the rebreathing of the anesthetic and oxygen. Curare, the first muscle relaxant, had been reported to be used in 1942 by Griffith and Johnson.(3) Academic leaders of the day cautioned that this drug should not be used during surgical procedures due to the inherit risks of paralysis.1 Nevertheless, over the next two decades muscle relaxants came into routine use and necessitated the use of endotracheal intubation, ventilators and recovery rooms. Although a training program in Anesthesiology had been initiated in 1927 by Ralph Waters at the University of Wisconsin, there were relatively few trained anesthesiologists when the United States entered World War II. It was clear during the war that there needed to be a great many more practitioners to meet the needs of the expanding number of surgical procedures. The quality and quantity of practitioners as well as the safety of anesthetic care was brought into question when Beecher and Todd presented the first anesthesia mortality study in 1952.(4) They demonstrated that death due to anesthesia occurred in 1:1, 560 surgical procedures. This led to a dramatic increase in the number of residency training programs for physicians as well as nurses in anesthesia and to the initiation of academic departments to foster the development of research programs.

In 1975, when I started medical school anesthesia machines had no required electronic monitors. Some had "bouncing ball" EKG scopes if patients were thought to have heart disease. Most machines also had FiO2 meters attached to the inspiratory limb of the circle system to ensure hypoxic mixtures of gases were not being given to the patient. Patients were monitored intraoperatively with a manual blood pressure cuff and a hand on the pulse if an EKG machine was not available. Between 1975 and 1980 EKG monitors became routine on every anesthesia machine and the first automatic noninvasive blood pressure (NIBP) devices were introduced. The 1980s was the decade of routine monitoring. Pulse oximetry, which was under development in the late 1970s, became a routine device by 1986 and was joined simultaneously with continuous carbon dioxide monitoring, capnography. Capnography had been routine in the Netherlands since the mid 1970s and was quickly adopted as one of the standard noninvasive monitors along with pulse oximetry, NIBP, EKG, FiO2 and temperature.(5) By the late 1980s anesthetic agent monitoring was also routine. The combination of these noninvasive physiologic monitors ensured ventilation, perfusion and oxygenation. Their use became a standard in 1987 and was credited with significantly reducing the anesthetic related mortality to the range of 1:500,000 by 1990. With the advent of invasive hemodynamic monitoring through the 1970s and 80s, a whole array of physiologic monitoring devices were readily available in the operating room to ensure that patients of any degree of illness or preexisting disease could be cared for adequately. During the same time frame, from the 1970s through the 1990s, anesthetic subspecialties developed in parallel to their surgical counterparts. Subspecialty fellowship training as well as certification followed the academic advances in research. The 1990s saw the adoption of transesophageal echocardiography for routine use in cardiac surgical cases, and also for diagnostic use in non-cardiac procedures in patients with serious cardiac disease. Over this twenty-year time period, surgical techniques dramatically expanded with advances in minimally invasive surgery, the routine use of microscopes and laproscopic procedures as well as digital radiologic imaging incorporated into the surgical process. Due to these minimally invasive and more precise surgical techniques patient length of stay in the hospital has been greatly reduced.

The operating room itself has not changed much in the past twenty years other than becoming increasingly crowded with a wide array of surgical devices and a much larger anesthesia machine with its attendant incorporated monitors. Anesthetic drugs have become as precise and targeted as have the surgical techniques. The first synthetic narcotic fentanyl introduced in the 1970s has been followed by sufentanyl, alfentanyl, and most recently, remifentanyl with a half-life of only seven minutes. Curare has been replaced by relaxants with fewer side-effects, more rapid onset and shorter duration of action. Total intravenous anesthesia with propofol and/or remifentanyl has allowed for profound analgesia and amnesia with rapid wake-up and minimal side effects. The laryngeal mask airway has replaced the anesthesia mask as a routine technique for patients not requiring endotrachael intubation.

The next 10 years will see the generalized deployment of comprehensive perioperative information systems. The current MorCARE system under development at the University of Michigan allows for all perioperative information and reference work to be immediately available at the anesthesia machine. As all of the information systems within the hospital coalesce we will see the final demise of the paper chart and the sooner, the better. On the immediate horizon in Surgery are the rapid advances in the robotic techniques. The incorporation of computers not only to the management of information, but to the management of the surgical and anesthetic techniques, foreshadows dramatic changes that will be seen in the next century.

2050 to 2100

Theodore Connor Tremper is born in 2050, the great-grandson of Kevin Keefe Tremper and seven-generations after R.H. Tremper, the surgical resident from Michigan. He was born in one of the newer labor and delivery family resorts initiated by Ritz Carlton in the late 2030s. Since labor could be initiated upon patient request without pain or discomfort, these resorts are able to book reservations many months in advance. Patients complete an online survey, which sorts them into ASA categories (still used). Based on their answers and previous medical information already in their online chart, the computer decides their ASA status (paper charts are now part of the Bentley Historical Library at the University of Michigan). The Ritz Carlton offers a wide variety of options from the Intimate Birth Package which can accommodate a family of 2-4 in a charming room with a fresh flowers, soft music and overstuffed furniture to the Family Reunion Birth Package which is set up in a theater type fashion for 20 of your closest family and friends to share in your experience. The Ritz Carlton offers a full array of decorating and catering options including Virtual Reality chambers where you can give birth anywhere in the world.

Much has changed in perioperative medicine over the last 50 years and many of those changes were initiated at the University of Michigan. The development of robotic surgery, not only expanded the capabilities of surgical procedures, but also dramatically effected the structure of what was once called Surgical Departments. The advanced technology applied to telemedicine at Robotic Procedure Centers (RPCs) required a different set of clinical specialists at the site of the patient encounter. The physicians at the RPC are not the individuals performing the actual procedure. Subspecialty Technical Surgical Groups are composed of surgeons located around the world in strategic time zones to allow procedures to be accomplished at any location, 24-hours a day. These global subspecialty surgical groups can provide their services at any time at thousands of interventional centers (hospitals or RPCs) throughout the world. The interventional centers are staffed by a new group of hospital specialist which grew out of the old Departments of Emergency Medicine, Trauma/Surgery, Anesthesiology and Critical Care. These practitioners prepare patients for the surgical procedures to be accomplished robotically by the remote specialists. They also supervise these robotic interventions and are prepared for emergency intervention should it be required. The high availability of cloned organs has made organ transplantation the most common surgical procedure. Because of the high cost of the robotic procedure suite by the year 2050, they are all being utilized 24-by-7 thereby requiring the growth of global alliances of surgeons by specific surgical procedure. The procedure rooms incorporated complete real-time body imaging, which allowed for high precision microsurgery. This imaging also completely replaced what used to be known as physiologic monitoring during anesthesia and surgery. On-line imaging of hemodynamic and metabolic function, ensures that total physiologic homeostasis is maintained during the procedures. The first global surgical alliance was initiated at the University of Michigan in 2018 by Lisa Colletti, MD, the first female Chair of Surgery.

Anesthetic and surgical preparations were changed dramatically by two innovations. The first was the development of PTIM Therapy (Pre-Traumatic Immune Manipulation). With the comprehensive understanding of the immune system and the ability to manipulate it pharmacologically, patients are pretreated prior to elective surgical procedures to prevent the harmful cascade of the inflammatory response and to optimize the recovery process. Healing from significant interventions is accomplished within days due to this therapy. The second innovation was Induced REM Anesthesia. Dr. Poe and Lydic demonstrated the first REM anesthetic in animals in 2016 also at the University of Michigan. Three years later human REM anesthetic was also conducted at Michigan. It had been long noted that during REM cycles muscles relax and the brain became active in a restorative way. Dr. Poe discovered of the a2 orexin receptor, which when activated produced a profound analgesia during REM sleep. The inclusion of induced REM during anesthesia allowed for the elimination of the use of traditional induction agents and the complete elimination of nausea and vomiting that had plagued anesthesia for over 150 years. The term "balanced-anesthesia" which used to mean the combination of narcotics, relaxants and nitrous oxide, now meant Xenon/Oxygen inhalation, a2 orexin with a low level of infusion of Neofentanyl, a specific agent for profound analgesia. Postoperative analgesia consisted of transdermal patches, which replaced the old intravenous PCA of the late 20th century. The patient's airway is secured with a device called the ETLMA. This is a combination of the old LMA airway and the endotrachael tube. It is inserted via digital image guidance after the induction of REM anesthesia. Each set of six surgical suites required two interventionalist physician teams as well as six biomedical information technologists and six interventionalist nurses.

Since recovery from anesthesia is nearly instantaneous, patients are observed and final scans are completed in the interventional suite and then discharged directly to the high intensity observation suite, the low intensity observation suite, or to home. Few elective procedures required more than an overnight stay including transplantation. Therefore, the majority of the hospitalized patients were those recovering from trauma. Hospitals have evolved to a combination of emergency departments, interventional suites and high intensity care suite (critical care units). Much of medical therapy is accomplished via telemedicine at the patients' home or office and therefore does not require large clinics or hospital floor beds as seen in the 20th century.

Theodore Connor Tremper initiated his training in Medicine at the University of Michigan's Virtual Medical School in 2075. His entrance requirements were the completion of the Microsoft-X Medicine Training Tutorial that had become the standard by 2065. Students interested in various aspects of medicine completed their knowledge-based and technical testing via programmed learning modules. These could be completed at any time and any location via the Michigan Microsoft Training Network. John Gates who focused much of the Microsoft Strategic Vision to Medicine and Education initiated this program. He was the grandson of the famous entrepreneur of the 20th century, Bill Gates. Susan Gates, John's cousin, was coincidentally the 18th President of the University of Michigan. It is also interesting to note that General Electric and Hewlett Packard are still competitors in the medical marketplace. Hospitalists still make telemedicine "rounds" at the University of Michigan on the Hewlett Service (named after Albion Walter Hewlett, the renowned Michigan internist and father of William Hewlett, co-founder of Hewlett Packard) which is now in the GE High Intensity Care Building. The following is the Table of Contents from Anesthesiology, Volume 187:12, December, 2099, (Special Memorial Edition printed on paper) which highlights landmark papers of the 21st century.(6)

(Commemorative Edition Available on Paper)
EDITORIAL

Hallmark Events in Anesthesia During the 21st Century
Theodore C. Tremper, Microsoft Professor of Anesthesia,
University of Michigan Medical School

CLASSIC PAPERS REVISITED

2025: Balanced-REM Anesthesia in Humans using a a2 orexin agonist.
2031: ETLMA Intubation Under MRI Guidance.
2038: Perioperative Modulation of Pro and anti-inflammatory Cytokines Accelerate Recovery from Surgical Intervention
2051: Neofentanyl-REM Balanced Anesthesia Improves Healing and Learning.
2065: Implantable Medical Information Chip: Failure Rate Reduce to 1:1,000,000
2070: Cost-effectiveness of Zero Gravity Ventilation

CASE REPORTS

Anesthesia for the First Spinal Cord Transplant
Anesthesia and Surgery on an Extraterrestrial from Logos
CORRESPONDENCE

Anesthesia Residents Fight to Retain the Twenty-Hour Work Week
Manual Endotracheal Intubation: A Lost Art

REFERENCES

1. Collins VJ. Principles of Anesthesiology, Second Ed., Chapter 1, The History of Anesthesiology, Lea and Febiges, Philadelphia, pgs 3-30, 1976.

2. Tremper, RH. Resident Thesis, University of Michigan, Department of Surgery, Class of 1875.

3. Griffith HR, Johnson GE. The Use of Curare in General Anesthesia. Anesthesiology 3:418, 1942.

4. Beecher H, Todd DP. A Study of the Deaths Associated with Anesthesia and Surgery. Annuals of Surgery 140:2, 1954.

5. Standards for Basic Anesthetic Monitoring (Approved by House of Delegates on October 21, 1986). Basics of Anesthesia, Third Ed. Stoelting RK and Miller RD, Churchill Livingstone, New York, pgs. 497-498, 1994.

6. Stoneham M. Personal Communication, 2002.

CHAPTER 7

THORACIC SURGERY

MARK D. IANNETTONI, M.D., M.B.A.

Introduction

John Alexander established the specialty of Thoracic Surgery at the University of Michigan in 1928, and started the first thoracic residency in the country. At that time, thoracic surgery was concerned mostly with the care and management of patients with tuberculosis and other infectious lung diseases. Since that time, the specialty has evolved into two basic divisions, general thoracic surgery and cardiac surgery. While these distinctions are strong in many university programs, the specialty is still a practice of both disciplines for approximately 80% of those involved with the specialty.

Scope of Practice

In general thoracic surgery the majority of patients have some type of end stage disease involving thoracic oncology or pulmonary or esophageal dysfunction. One of the more rapidly expanding fields is minimally invasive surgery (MIS) for both diagnosis as well as treatment. The greatest advancements in general thoracic surgery have come from improvements in diagnostic imaging allowing directed diagnostic or therapeutic operative techniques utilizing MIS.

Diagnostic Techniques
Endoscopy

Endoscopy of the aerodigestive tract is essential for evaluation of esophageal or pulmonary malignancy; in the past this modality was limited to direct visualization and biopsy of luminal disease. Recently, the addition of ultrasonography has allowed a more detailed appreciation of the anatomy of the esophageal wall as well as allowing staging by identification and biopsy of nodes with in the mediastinum or the upper abdomen. Biopsy can be accomplished from either the trachea or esophagus.(1)

Bronchoscopic ultrasound combined with needle aspiration has been shown to be as sensitive and specific as mediastinoscopy for the diagnosis and staging of patients with pulmonary malignancy.(2) This approach has markedly reduced the number of medastinoscopies required and has resulted in improvements in stage-directed therapy.

Similarly, endoscopic ultrasound (EUS) for esophageal cancer has resulted in better staging of esophageal malignancy. This modality allows the evaluation of involved lymph nodes and accurately stages the depth of penetration of the wall of the esophagus and involvement of adjacent structures.(3) For patients that undergo preoperative chemotherapy and radiation therapy, post-treatment EUS can be used to determine if clinical response has occurred. At present, it appears that EUS is more accurate than CT for these determinations. EUS has also recently been used as an adjunct treatment method for mediastinal masses and cysts and may be the procedure of choice in the future for bronchogenic or esophageal duplication cysts.(4)

Computerized Tomography

Computerized tomography has been utilized extensively in thoracic surgery as the imaging procedure of choice. However, it has not been cost effective to use this modality as a method of screening. Currently, there are rapid scanners with the ability to perform total body CT in less than a minute that also allow digital archiving of imaging data. This potential has resulted in the use of CT as a screening modality and studies are currently underway to prove its cost effectiveness as well as its clinical benefit for this purpose.

Positron Emission Testing

One of the major diagnostic advances in imaging for thoracic surgery has been the development of positron emission testing (PET). Prior to PET scanning a 30-40% rate of exploratory thoracotomy with findings of benign disease was acceptable. With PET scanning, patients with a lesion greater than 8 mm which does not fit the usual profile for malignancy, and have no old radiographs, can undergo PET scanning as part of their evaluation and treatment.(5) PET evaluation has eliminated the requirement for needle biopsy or thoracotomy in patients with a negative scan. The PET scan has also allowed patients with marginal function to become candidates for resection or observation rather than undergoing an exploratory thoracotomy.(6, 7)

Technical Advances
Minimally Invasive Surgery

Minimally invasive surgery (MIS) has resulted in improvements in patient care by allowing similar operations to be done with faster recovery and a more rapid return to work, as well as decreasing hospital stay. The major problem with MIS was assuring that the same operation was done via the ports as was being done open. Initially, the results with laparoscopic and thoracoscopic surgery were not equivalent to open operative results and procedures such as laparoscopic Nissen fundoplication and thoracoscopic wedge resection resulted in less than stellar results. After an initial learning curve was overcome, the procedures have now become the preference for many patients.

The use of MIS for esophageal disease has resulted in a more liberal use of fundoplication since the procedure is performed via the laparoscope, and can be more cost effective than the use of proton pump inhibitors long term.

MIS has all but eliminated the need for thoracotomy for patients with achalasia. The use of botulinum toxin injections for temporary relief has dramatically decreased, and patients who fail initial balloon dilation are referred for MIS as their next step in treatment. While long-term results remain to be confirmed, initial results appear to be equal to the open procedure. This treatment will hopefully limit the number of patients seen with end stage disease who require esophagectomy, since patients are being referred earlier.

Transhiatal esophagectomy has gained worldwide acceptance. The use of MIS for esophageal resection is currently undergoing evaluation at a few select centers.(8) The technical aspects of the operations are similar. With time, MIS esophagectomy may evolve into an outpatient operation or short stay procedure with better postoperative results.

MIS for lung disease has also improved patient care. The ability to perform any thoracic procedure without a thoracotomy significantly impacts the patient's overall recovery, hospital stay, and in some cases, ability to receive treatment at all. Many patients with marginal pulmonary function were denied surgery in the past because they were unable to withstand a thoracotomy. With the use of thoracoscopy some of these patients are not only able to tolerate the procedure, they can also have a lesser operation with the same 5-year survival. Limited or nonanatomic resection has received criticism because of fears of a high local recurrence rate and for not being a complete cancer operation. Recent studies have shown that 5-year survival is the same when compared stage for stage.(9) Although thoracoscopy has resulted in improved patient access, long-term pain syndromes are unchanged, with 3% of patients complaining of long-term post thoracotomy pain.(10)

One of the benefits of MIS is a decreased hospitalization for patients who require wedge resection. Investigators have recently presented and published the first experience with outpatient thoracoscopy for pulmonary wedge resection. They have shown that it is possible to provide this service to over 90% of patients with no mortality or increase in morbidity.(11)

Photodynamic Therapy

With an increase in the total number of patients with esophageal cancer, there has also been an increase in the number of patients with inoperable disease. Surgeons have attempted to identify new means of palliation for patients who are not surgical candidates. The use of photodynamic therapy is one way to palliate patients without surgery. The availability of a photosensitizing agent activated by monochromatic light utilizing a non-thermal LASER has resulted in an outpatient therapy that improves dysphagia almost immediately. However, the current agents are relatively expensive, limiting their use on a more liberal basis.

A current interest in this modality involves its use for Barrett's esophagus and with the ability to remove abnormal tissue permanently, thereby eliminating it as a precursor for cancer. Although studies suggest that this may be a feasible method of treatment for many patients the long-term results need to be assessed.(12, 13, 14)

The use of photodynamic therapy for airway obstruction has not been as gratifying. Although the airway can be cleared of tumor, phototherapy is not durable and requires an inpatient stay. Clinical results with thermal LASER have been almost equal and are considerably less expensive.

Stents

All too frequently surgeons see patients in whom tumors result in airway or esophageal obstruction, with a cause that is not endoluminal. These patients had few therapeutic alternatives in the past; the advent of expandable metallic stents has significantly improved palliation and lifestyle in many patients for the short term.(15, 16) Stents are a poor choice for long term use due to significant complications such as overgrowth with granulation tissue, obstruction or erosion.(17, 18, 19)

Future Directions
Lobar Transplantation

One of the most exciting frontiers in thoracic surgery is that of living related lung transplantation. With the paucity of donors and the lack of currently available support devices, a few centers have examined the possibility of lobar transplantation. Initially, this resulted in a higher morbidity and mortality in the donor population than was acceptable but with further experience complications have improved. The results for the recipients have not been as good as for cadaveric transplantation. As with any new procedure the learning curve is steep and should be accomplished with the same results as currently published for cadaveric transplantation.(20)

Gene Directed Therapy

A major goal of thoracic research programs has been identification of genes that play a role in the development and progression of esophageal and lung adenocarcinomas. Over the past decade, many translational studies using surgically obtained tissues and established cell lines have focused on these important cancers with the goal of obtaining a greater understanding of disease and potentially new avenues for early detection or treatment. Two research areas deserve particular attention and are described below.

Detection of Novel Gene Amplification Events in Esophageal Adenocarcinomas

In addition to tumor samples, normal squamous mucosa as well as Barrett's meta-plasia may be obtained from patients undergoing esophagectomy for cancer. These samples provide control tissue for each patient to examine whether gene alterations present in the patient's tumor also are present in the premalignant Barrett's metaplasia. A large number of esophageal adenocarcinomas, Barrett's metaplasia, and normal squamous mucosa have been examined using the genome scanning technique of 2D analysis of restriction fragments which has resulted in the identification of novel gene amplification events in this tumor type.(20) Gene amplification can result in a selective increase in the number of copies of a particular gene. Amplification may provide a powerful selective advantage if genes involved in growth control or differentiation are affected. As one example, the amplicon identified at chromosome 8p22-23 results in the over expression of cathepsin B, a gene involved in invasion and metastasis.

Using quantitative polymerase chain reaction, one may also examine the potential over expression of mRNA for 12 uncharacterized ESTs and two known genes located within the "minimal region of common amplification" for the 8p22-23 amplicon. In addition to cathepsin B, only one of the 11 ESTs was found to be highly over expressed at the mRNA level in the esophageal adenocarcinomas demonstrating 8p22-23 amplification. This EST was extensively analyzed for sequence similarity and found to be homologous to the 3' region of the zinc-finger transcription factor GATA-4. High levels of the GATA-4 protein were also present in the tumors demonstrating amplification of 8p22 but not in nonamplified tumors.(21)

The genome scanning approach is ideally suited for the identification of DNA amplification events without the need for knowing, a priori, the identity of the genes being examined. DNA gels of esophageal adenocarcinomas reveal over 2500 individual DNA fragments per combination of restriction enzymes. Using this approach investigators have recently reported (22) the amplification of the cyclin E gene in esophageal adenocarcinomas. An important component of these studies is the ability to also examine the premalignant, dysplastic Barrett's metaplasia from these patients. Cyclin E amplification may precede adenocarcinoma development. These studies hold significant potential to identify important cancer-related genes in these tumors and to potentially delineate strategies for early cancer detection for patients with Barrett's metaplasia.

Gene and Protein Expression Profiles Predictive of Patient Survival in Stage I Lung Adenocarcinomas

Recent advances in technology have now allowed the analysis of thousands of genes and hundreds of proteins simultaneously. Using an mRNA and protein profiling approach a current research effort is to determine whether these profiles can identify high-risk patients who have early stage lung cancer. A series of 90 lung adenocarcinomas and ten uninvolved lung samples were examined for protein expression using 2-D polyacrylamide gel electrophoresis (2-D PAGE) and candidate proteins analyzed using matrix-assisted laser desorption/ionization mass spectrometry (MALDI-MS). A total of 820 individual protein spots were quantified for each sample. These same tumors samples were also analyzed using oligonucleotide microarrays and expression of 6800 genes were examined. Fifty protein spots and over 300 genes were found to be significantly correlated with patient survival using Cox proportional hazards regression analysis. Expression profiles for the 20 proteins, or the 50 top genes, that were most significantly correlated with survival were used to create a risk index using a leave-one-out, cross-validation method. Separate high and low risk groups were identified among patients with stage I lung adenocarcinoma that differed significantly in patient survival.

Defining genes or proteins that identify patients with early stage lung cancer who are at high-risk is expected to lead to new clinical trials to provide these patients with adjuvant therapy in addition to surgical resection. These studies have already identified genes and proteins previously characterized as involved in lung cancer, but also many new candidates with the potential for identifying new avenues for intervention or early detection.

Artificial Lung

Devices and techniques used for cardiopulmonary bypass during surgery have been applied for the past thirty years for prolonged cardiopulmonary support. Such prolonged support, commonly referred to as "extracorporeal membrane oxygenation" (ECMO), is used with a few thousand patients each year, mostly neonatal or pediatric patients with impaired cardiac and/or pulmonary function. The conditions seen in the majority of these patients (e.g., congenital diaphragmatic hernia, meconium aspiration syndrome) resolve with or without medical/surgical intervention in a relatively short time; the duration of ECMO support is typically less than one week, with a few patients supported for more than one month. Although the use of ECMO in adults has grown in the past several years, the duration of support required for indicated conditions in adults is much longer than in the neonatal/pediatric population; the complications associated with such extended therapy have prompted the development of alternative means of support.

Several complications arise when ECMO is applied for extended periods. Blood/surface interactions that are not significant in a few hours during bypass surgery become problematic over several days or weeks of prolonged support. Despite anticoagulation protocols, microembolism and gross thrombus formation can occur. Mechanical effects of blood pumps cause destruction of blood cells and activation of platelets.

Recently, attempts have been made to decrease the surface area of an ECMO system by building an integrated pump/oxygenator. These devices may find applications in situations where ECMO is used today and where both cardiac and pulmonary support are required; however, the inclusion of a pump in these systems leads to significant drawbacks for their use in extended pulmonary support.

Various approaches have been taken to provide prolonged pulmonary support. The Intravenacaval Oxygenator (IVOX®) (23) is a catheter that is used to position a bundle of gas exchange fibers roughly 50 cm in length and 5 - 10 mm in diameter into the vena cava through either a femoral or jugular venotomy. The bundle of fibers is intended to unravel in the vena cava and provide gas exchange across the fibers without significantly impeding blood flow. The appeal of this approach is the simple insertion of the device. However, the IVOX® is capable of providing less than 1/3 of the gas exchange needs of an adult, so its potential application is limited. Several design changes have been made over the past several years in order to make an intravenacaval device with more efficient gas transfer, but there is currently no such device available that can support the gas exchange needs of an adult.

Another approach to extended pulmonary support is the paracorporeal artificial lung (PAL). The PAL was designed to be analogous to the ventricular assist device (VAD) for cardiac support, as the PAL is also attached directly to the heart and the surrounding vessels via end-to-side anastomoses using large diameter synthetic grafts. Typical attachment modes involve placement of the device either in parallel with the native lungs (pulmonary artery to left atrium) or in series with the lungs (proximal to distal pulmonary artery, with a snare between the anastomoses to divert flow through the PAL). The PAL conduits are tunneled, and the device is secured to the patient's chest. A source of oxygen is connected to the device, and blood flow, oxygenation and CO_2 removal are monitored continuously. The PAL is similar in concept to the membrane oxygenator used in a heart/lung machine. However, the PAL required substantial modifications to the standard oxygenator design to permit its use without an auxiliary pump and to make it suitable for prolonged use.

Early attempts at the PAL concept involved attaching a commercial blood oxygenator to the heart. The right heart failed very quickly, due to the increased impedance to blood flow of the oxygenator compared to the native lungs. The oxygenator design was modified over several iterations to decrease the resistance to blood flow; when resistance had been decreased nearly a factor of ten, the right heart was able to tolerate the presence of the device for several hours without failure when the device was placed in parallel with the native lungs. However, right heart failure was still a problem when the device was placed PA-PA. A compliant chamber was added to the inlet of the PAL to compensate for the extra work required by the heart to pump blood into the rigid PAL container. After compliance was added, the right heart tolerated the device, and work required by the heart decreased.(24, 25, 26, 27)

It has yet to be determined the best mode of attachment for the device. The PA-PA (series) attachment allows perfusion of the lungs with oxygenated blood and maintains the filtering and endocrine functions of the lungs, but the work of the heart is increased. The PA-LA attachment permits competitive flow between the native lungs and the artificial device, and the work required by the heart is decreased. However, microemboli formation in the device must be carefully avoided.

Potential applications of the PAL include bridge to lung transplant for patients with end stage lung disease of rapid onset. Another use for this device could be for patients who require ventilatory support for chronic disease. The artificial lung could be used to allow these people to be removed from the ventilator much as an artificial heart allows separation from ECMO.

Robotics

The technological advances that have taken place over the past few years have resulted in revolutionary new methods of patient care. Robotics, originally utilized to improve quality control and production, have been applied to medicine recently. This concept, originally developed by the military, was intended to allow for battlefield treatment of casualties from a remote location. This operation-at-a-distance would avoid the need for a skilled professional to be at the front lines while still providing expert technical care for patients.

The current use of the robotic system in thoracic surgery is limited but is being evaluated for lung resection, esophageal surgery, and the treatment of mediastinal disease.

Patient Care

The computer age has resulted in an explosion of access to medical knowledge. This access has resulted in a more educated and informed patient. Many patients now present with results and articles, and other options from the Internet. Web sites for education and advertisement have resulted in expanding the knowledge base of both the patient and the physician.

One of the major initiatives of the Society of Thoracic Surgeons (STS) has been the Cardiothoracic Surgeons Network (CTSNET). This site lists all the major topics involved with thoracic surgery, web broadcasts of major meetings and is now involved with a web based patient information system. Already established is a resident database for case logs as well as an online education guide for our thoracic residents. Also available for patients is a listing of all board-certified members and physician profiles for patients with specialty directories and links to other informational web sites.

This service allows patients to obtain up to date information and treatment options. In the planning stages are listings of cooperative trials, which will also list eligibility criteria for patients to aid in their care as well as a site for physician education.

In the future, teleconferencing will allow for outside physicians to share patient information and permit options for care and consultation from remote sites. The patient would be able to telenet with the physician of their choice from any location with the aid of a local physician providing further testing and data submission. One of the major obstacles to this form of treatment will be the protection of information across the Internet as well as data archiving. These goals will require controlled access and secure data lines.

Centers of Excellence

One of the most controversial topics in thoracic surgery is the concept of centers of excellence. This designation would distinguish a program or institution as being superior to another because of volume, results, and experience. The implications of the stature are obvious both from an educational and a financial viewpoint. This type of designation has been fostered by many of the major insurance companies, citing surgical data that shows support for specialty training and volume.

A number of studies have clearly shown that the results for esophagectomy are directly related to the volume of cases performed. These data lend support for centers of excellence for this type of procedure. This system has been used in Canada and Japan with great success. Studies have also demonstrated that it is important not only where the procedure is done but also by whom. For lung resection, morbidity and mortality was significantly reduced when operations were performed by specialists rather than by generalist with no specialty training. Although such a policy results in limited access, it does result better patient care as well as more cost effective medicine.

Although only limited data are available for patient outcomes with respect to these types of questions, the Society of Thoracic Surgery is currently sponsoring national database requirements for all members to collect outcomes data. This mandate will allow a better analysis of factors to improve patients care and allow a platform for cooperative trials and critical pathways to unify patient care. This central database repository will also allow comparison of patient outcomes, and individual results can be analyzed, with risk-adjustment.

REFERENCES

1. Wallace MB, Sivestri GA, Sahai AV, Hawes RH, Hoffman BJ, Durkalski V, Hennesey WS, Reed CE. Endoscopic ultrasound-guided fine needle aspiration for staging patients with carcinoma of the lung. Ann Thorac Surg 2001 Dec; 72(6):1861-7

2. Lau CL, Harpole DH Jr, Patz E. Staging techniques for lung cancer. Chest Surg Clin N Am. 2000 Nov; 10(4):781-801. Review

3. Rice TW. Clinical staging of esophageal carcinoma. CT, EUS, and PET. Chest Surg Clin N Am. 2000 Aug; 10(3):471-85. Review

4. Pedersen BH, Vilmann P, Milman N, Folke K, Hancke S. Endoscopic ultrasonography with guided fine needle aspiration biopsy of a mediastinal mass lesion. Acta Radiol 1995 May;36(3):326-8

5. Hicks RJ Kalff V, MacManus MP, Ware RE, Hogg A, McKenzie-Ball DL. (18) F-FDG PET provides high-impact and powerful prognostic staging newly diagnosed non-small cell lung cancer. J Nucl Med. 2001 Noc;42(11):1596-604

6. Gupta NC, Tamim WJ, Graeber GG, Bishop HA, Hobbs GR. Mediastinal lymph node sampling following positron emission fluorodeoxyglucose imaging in lung cancer staging. Chest 2001 Aug; 120(2):521-7

7. Dunagan D, Chin R Jr, McCain T, Case L, Harkness B, Oaks. Staging by positron emission tomography predicts survival in non-small cell lung cancer. Chest 2001 Feb;119(2):333-9

8. Luketich JD, Fernando HC, Christie NA, Buenaventura PO, Keenan RJ, Ikramuddin S, Schauer PR. Outcomes after minimally invasive esophagomyotomy. Ann Thorac Surg. 2001 Dec;72(6):1909-12; discussion 1912-3

9. Ginsberg RJ, Rubinstein LV. Randomized trial of lobectomy versus limited resection for T1 N0 non-small cell lung cancer. Lung Cancer Study Group. Ann Thorac Surg 1995 Sep;60(3):615-22:discussion 622-3

10. Landreneau RJ, Wiechmann RJ, Hazelrigg SR, Mack MJ, Keenan RJ, Ferson PF. Effect of minimally invasive thoracic surgical approaches on acute and chronic postoperative pain. Chest Surg Clin N Am. 1998 Nov;8(4):891-906. Review

11. Chang AC, Yee J, Iannettoni MD, Orringer MB. Diagnostic Thoracoscopy Lung Biopsy: An Outpatient Experience. Submitted to Society of Thoracic Surgeons August 2001.Presented at AATS

12. Panjehpour M, Overholt BF, Haydek JM, Lee SG. Results of photodynamic therapy for ablation of dysplasia and early cancer in Barrett's esophagus and effect of oral steroids on stricture formation. AM J Gastroenterol 2000 Sep;95(9):2177-84

13. Overholt BF, Panjehpour M. Photodynamic therapy in the management of Barrett's esophagus with dysplasia. J Gastrointest Surg 2000 Mar-Apr;4(2):129-30. Review

14. Overholt BF, Panjehpour M, Haydek JM. Photodynamic therapy for Barrett's esophagus: follow-up in 100 patients. Gastrointest Endosc. 1999 Jan;49(1):1-7

15. Mosca F, Stracqualursi A, Portale TR, Consoli A, Latteri S. Palliative treatment of malignant esophageal stenosis: the role of self-expanding stent endoscopic implantation. Dis Esophagus 2000;13(4):301-4

16. Madden BP, Stamenkovic SA, Mitchell P. Covered expandable tracheal stents in the management of benign tracheal granulation tissue formation. Ann Thorac Surg 2000 Oct: 70(4):1191-3

17. Ackroyd R, Watson DI, Devitt PG, Jamieson GG. Expandable metallic stents should not be used in the treatment of benign esophageal strictures. J Gastroenterol Hepatol 2001 Apr;16(4):484-7

18. Cordero JA Jr, Moores DW. Self-expanding esophageal metallic stents in the treatment of esophageal obstruction. Am Surg 2000 Oct;66(10):956-8; discussion 958-9

19. Wang MQ, Sze DY, Wang ZP, Wang ZQ, Gao YA, Dake MD. Delayed complications after esophageal stent placement for treatment of malignant esophageal obstructions and esophagorespiratory fistulas. J Vasc Interv Radiol 2001 Apr;12(4):465-74

20. Camarow, A. Transplant. US News and World Report July 23, 2001

21. Hughes SJ, Glover TW, Zhu XX, Kuick R, Thoraval D, Orringer MB, Beer DG, Hanash S. (1998) A novel amplicon at 8p22-23 results in overexpression of cathepsin B in esophageal adenocarcinoma. Proc Natl Acad Sci (USA) 12410-12415

22. Lin L, Aggarwal S, Glover TW, Orringer, MB, Hanash S, Beer DG. A minimal critical region of the 8p22-23 amplicon in esophageal adenocarcinomas defined using STS-amplification mapping and quatitative PCR includes the GATA-4 gene. Cancer Res. 60:1341-1347, 2000

23. Lin L, Prescott MS, Zhu Z, Singh P, Chun SY, Kuick RD, Hanash S, Orringer, MB, Glover TW, Beer DG. Identification and characterization of a 19q12 amplicon in esophageal adenocarcinomas reveals cyclin E as the best candidate gene for this amplicon. Cancer Res.60:7021-7027, 2000

24. Mortensen JD, Berry G. Conceptual and design features of a practical, clinically effective intravenous mechanical blood oxygen/carbon dioxide exchange device (IVOX). Int J Artif Organs. 1989 Jun;12(6):384-9

25. Lynch WR, Montoya JP, Brant DO, Schreiner RJ, Iannettoni MD, Bartlett RH. Hemodynamic effect of a low-resistance artificial lung in series with the native lungs of sheep. Ann Thorac Surg. 2000 Feb;69(2):351-6

26. Lick SD, Zwischenberger JB, Wang D, Deyo DJ, Alpard SK, Chambers SD. Improved right heart function with a compliant inflow artificial lung in series with the pulmonary circulation. Ann Thorac Surg. 2001 Sep;72(3):899-904

27. Haft JW, Montoya P, Alnajjar O, Posner SR, Bull JL, Iannettoni MD, Bartlett RH, Hirschl RB. An artificial lung reduces pulmonary impedance and improves right ventricular efficiency in pulmonary hypertension. J Thorac Cardiovasc Surg. 2001 Dec;122(6):1094-1001

CHAPTER 8

CARDIAC SURGERY

RICHARD N. PIERSON III, M.D., FRANK G. SCHOLL, M.D.

Introduction

Cardiac surgery has achieved remarkable successes over the past half-century. Cardiopulmonary bypass, myocardial protection, valve repair and replacement, surgical revascularization of ischemic myocardium, correction of complex congenital cardiac anomalies, heart and heart-lung transplantation, and mechanical cardiac assist and replacement are but a few of our most visible triumphs. Indeed not only are these therapies now available, but most are now almost routine, relatively safe, and indeed taken for granted.

Despite these triumphs, the new millennium finds cardiac surgeons under siege. Referred patients tend to be older and sicker, requiring more time, effort, and skill than in the past to achieve excellent outcomes, which are now expected, and often publicly reported. Professional reimbursement for the most common "non-cognitive" therapeutic interventions (as cardiac surgical procedures are euphemistically considered) continues to fall at approximately 10% per year. Cardiopulmonary bypass, the traditional platform around which the field grew, is associated with long-term neurocognitive impairment.[1] Increasingly we compete for patients with our traditional source of referrals as diagnostic cardiologists have developed increasingly effective percutaneous interventional approaches. Evidence that stents coated with anti-proliferative material such as rapamycin decrease the incidence of in-stent restenosis heralds further inroads by the interventional cardiologist into the shrinking population of patients referred for traditional surgical coronary revascularization.[2, 3] Now we are only asked to consider for surgery those patients who are either not candidates for percutaneous interventions, have failed this approach, or are recognized to have serious concomitant valvular pathology. Meanwhile the public perceives cardiac surgeons as emblematic of a medical profession increasingly driven by self-interest and avarice, and insufficiently attentive to the emotional needs of the patient. Given these pressures, it is not surprising that fewer top medical graduates choose the arduous seven or eight year residency training necessary to become certified in cardiac surgery; a rising number of cardiothoracic program slots have gone unfilled in recent matches.[4]

In this chapter we will explore the technological and logistical changes that we expect to occur in the coming decades. From this evolving foundation we will explore how evolutionary and revolutionary changes in philosophy, tools, and procedures may be brought to bear to return cardiac surgery to a central, positive, and respected role in the medical community.

Intra-operative Perfusion Technology

Important opportunities for improvement exist in our understanding of the inflammatory response to cardiopulmonary bypass, management of ischemia/reperfusion injury, and regulation of the coagulation system. Based on several decades of intense scientific scrutiny in these areas, complement inhibitors, cytokine and adhesion molecule blockers, pathway-specific anticoagulants, lazaroids, and other anti-inflammatory agents have all recently cleared clinical safety hurdles and are being tested for efficacy in various pathologic states. Coordination of these pharmacologic measures will allow the surgeon to more tightly regulate the body's innate immune response to surgical tissue injury and circulatory support. As our ability improves to limit the "collateral damage" currently associated with our interventions, the most important barrier to surgical referral will recede.

Approaches currently used clinically to measure the adequacy of tissue perfusion are primitive, and ignore the variable consequences of extracorporeal support in different tissue beds. Measurement of pharyngeal, gastric, and rectal mucosal pH, central venous oxygen content, and arterial blood chemistry will evolve to more sophisticated non-invasive devices to measure cellular metabolism, perhaps based on intraoperative magnetic resonance imaging of brain, skeletal muscle, and intraabdominal viscera. Once perturbations in cellular physiology can be identified during the operation, interventions can be developed to prevent adverse outcomes, rather than simply managing their consequences.

Technical advances in cardiopulmonary bypass will continue to provide safer, more biocompatible systems and circuits. Based on extensive work showing the pro-coagulant and pro-inflammatory consequences on blood after exposure to tubing and pump materials, heparin-coated circuits are now standard. Further advances at the interface between cellular biology and bioengineering are likely to deliver further improvements in biocompatibility of perfusion equipment in the coming decades.

Early adoption is likely for smaller circuits situated in closer proximity to the patient. These minimize both hemodilution and blood contact surface area. Prototypes incorporate sophisticated probes and self-regulating switches to eliminate air and particulates without interrupting pump function. Although this approach requires that the surgeon and perfusionist fundamentally change their strategies and interactions, if devices based on this type of automated system prove reliable and applicable in general practice, they may decrease the need for human intervention and thus "pilot error". Rapid continuous retrieval and washing of blood scavenged from the surgical field using cell-saver technology is an important adjunctive technique to limit the inflammatory response, prevent microembolization, and reduce transfusion requirements. A new generation of "smart" cannulas is being developed which incorporates filters or other features to limit particulate or gaseous embolization. Access catheter and cannula systems which eliminate the need for purse string sutures, and which automatically seal the insertion site upon removal, are likely to be in use over the next decade. Designs which eliminate current concerns about causing arterial dissection could facilitate safe institution of circulatory support within the chest via minimal access ports. Adjunctive techniques such as transesophageal echocardiography and epiaortic scanning to select cannulation sites will probably replace the relatively insensitive tactile and visual information available to the surgeon through the open chest.

Percutaneous coaxial devices to provide right heart support for complicated "off-pump" cases may improve safety and broaden the application of this technique. In addition, thin-walled high-flow catheters are now available which allow partial left heart support from groin access: oxygenated blood retrieved via a venous catheter placed across the interatrial septum into the left atrium is perfused into a femoral artery. These devices could greatly simplify stabilization and management of most patients with cardiogenic shock without the need for major surgery to institute effective support. Availability of these devices in the community will enhance the efficacy of the regional "hub and spoke" mechanical support systems pioneered by Oz and colleagues in the New York area.(5)

Coronary Revascularization

The appropriate objective of myocardial revascularization by any approach is, and should remain, complete, durable revascularization of all ischemic regions. The standards set by surgical therapy are now approached by aggressive interventionalists for a growing minority of patients. To compete effectively with them cardiac surgeons need to develop safe, individually tailored approaches that are not only "minimal access", but more importantly they should minimally perturb the patient's physiology. The validity of this paradigm is supported by the rapid adoption of "off-pump" coronary revascularization. Further, we will need to improve upon and rigorously document short and long-term outcomes, while keeping cost-effectiveness in view.

One alternative to our current dependence on cardiology is to compete effectively for primary referrals from general practitioners and patients. This may require us to master diagnostic algorithms, add percutaneous interventions to our armamentarium, and overcome substantial credentialing hurdles along the way. An intermediate -- and politically more tenable -- approach is to develop collaborative revascularization approaches jointly with the cardiologist. One might envision a hybrid "minimal access" technique, with endoscopic left internal mammary harvest and robotic "off-pump" anastomosis to the left anterior descending artery, followed by deployment of rapamycin coated stents in other coronary distributions, all during the same anesthetic. This approach might yield results comparable to surgical revascularization for patients who choose a "minimally invasive" solution. In any event percutaneous intervention technology needs to become part of the cardiac surgical curriculum, so that we better understand its capabilities and limitations, and can incorporate derivative technologies when it is in our patient's best interest.

The application of new technology to "old" operations will grow significantly over the next decade. Harvesting of arterial and venous conduits using minimal access techniques and the use of the harmonic scalpel have been shown to provide excellent quality conduit while limiting the "collateral damage" of a large skin incision, suture and/or clip materials and thermal injury to the conduit and surrounding tissues from traditional electrocautery. The use of all arterial grafting is being re-evaluated in an effort to re-define the historical standard surgical graft patency rates documented for vein grafts. Techniques to procure and construct composite radial and mammary grafts continue to be refined; unfortunately careful, complete follow-up is not typically available. The first generation of sutureless devices for creating proximal anastomoses during coronary artery bypass grafting has recently received final FDA approval. These devices appear to provide safe, rapid, high quality anastomoses. Because they decrease or eliminate manipulation and clamping of the aorta, atheroembolism and its neurologic consequences may be significantly reduced. Sutureless magnetic connectors for both proximal and distal anastomoses are in pre-clinical testing, and are just one example of revolutionary approaches that may prove superior to conventional suturing.

Endoscopic robot-assisted mammary harvesting and anastomoses of the left internal mammary to the left anterior descending artery have been accomplished using "minimal access" techniques. Using current technology, a single vessel LIMA-to-LAD typically takes four to six hours, has a significant learning curve, and inferior immediate and short term patency. Wide application must wait until the technology evolves to enable grafting of the circumflex and right coronary distributions, with equal or superior anastomotic patency and patient safety. This said, improvements in robotics will soon allow surgeons real time "haptic" (tactile) feedback. Improved three-dimensional visualization, synchronized instrument motion timed to the cardiac cycle, and automatic sutureless devices for proximal and distal anastomoses are examples of emerging technologies that offer promising solutions to the current obstacles.

It is likely that we will soon be able to use computer models to optimize graft orientation and anastamotic strategies before and during surgery. Based on 3D angiography or MRI data entered into high-speed computers, algorithms could be developed to account for individual patient cardiac geometry and coronary physiology and flow patterns. Based on modeling idiosyncratic flow characteristics, including effects of competitive flow, turbulence, and sequential versus individual touchdown grafting strategies, computer modeling might even be able to predict, intra-operatively, which of several strategies for deploying an individual patient's available conduit is likely to yield optimal graft flows and, presumably, long-term patency rates. Coupled with reliable real time intraoperative feedback regarding actual graft flow characteristics, for the first time we might be able to completely avoid early technical failures, and significantly raise the standard for clinical practice.

Valvular Heart Disease

Prosthetic valves and valve repair techniques continue to evolve. Preoperative high-speed MRI and transesophageal echocardiography can specifically identify lesions, and precisely define possible corrective approaches, while on-line computer modeling is being developed to predict biomechanical and physiologic results with various alternative interventions. Near real-time 3-dimensional TEE is already in early clinical use. As highly accurate diagnostic and anatomic descriptions of the valves become available intra-operatively, communication between surgeon, anesthesiologist, and echocardiographer will become increasingly important as more complex pathology and associated repairs are assessed. This interaction will be greatly facilitated by ready accessibility of digital information for expert interpretation without requiring physical presence of the cardiologist in the operating room.

Current approaches to valvular heart surgery depend on accurately placing many individual sutures and on securely tying multiple knots. Driven primarily by minimal access considerations, and particularly by the technical challenges of "tying knots in a vase with chopsticks", valve replacement strategies are evolving toward "sutureless" or "self-sewing" valves. Alternatively "self-tying" sutures made using Nitenol® technology may preserve the advantages of individual suture placement when the geometry of the patient is not readily amenable to insertion of prefabricated prostheses. While the specter of catheter-based valve repair or even replacement seems remote, it is certain that exploratory efforts will continue.

Increased efforts to utilize autologous tissues wherever possible have led to renewed interest in the Ross procedure for aortic valve replacement. This entails transplanting the patient's pulmonic valve to the aortic position, and replacing the pulmonic valve with a prosthesis, usually with an allogeneic homograft. An alternative novel technique is being developed to construct the aortic valve prosthesis from the autologous main pulmonary artery, which can then be replaced with a simple tube graft. This approach would avoid the risk of later degeneration or calcification of the allograft valve. Incremental improvements in valve scaffold design and construction are occurring in parallel with cellular biologic approaches to facilitate immigration and normal differentiation of native cells into xenogeneic or synthetic valve templates. Tissue engineers are also pursuing various approaches to "grow" valves from the patients own pleuripotent "stem" cells. However de novo growth of functional valves (let alone whole organs) entirely from an individual patient's own cells seems far off.

Robotically-based minimal access approaches are already being used to repair major intracardiac pathology. Small series of mitral valve repairs and ASD closures have been reported, demonstrating that this technology can be successfully applied, at least in carefully selected patients by experienced practitioners. If early results from pioneering centers are confirmed elsewhere and prove easily taught, the next decade will see broad dissemination of this technology, driven by patient demand and hospital marketing perhaps even more than surgeon preference.

Atrial Arrhythmia Surgery

The introduction of the "Maze" operation allowed cardiac surgeons to cure atrial fibrillation in nearly all patients.(6) Linear lesion patterns are created by sharp dissection, electrically isolating reentrant foci in the pulmonary veins and left and right atrial appendages; the edges of the lesions and various incisions connecting them are then sewn back together. However the magnitude of the operation, the requirement for cardiopulmonary bypass, and clotting and bleeding problems attendant to multiple intra-cardiac suture lines have proven a significant barrier to wide application. Consequently techniques for closed heart, "off-pump" ablation of atrial reentrant pathways have been introduced. Hyperthemia, crooprobe, laser, microwave, and ultrasonic energy sources are all being developed and adapted for minimal access approaches. If cure rates approaching 100% can be accomplished using "minimal access" techniques without cardiopulmonary bypass, the surgeon should be able to compete successfully with catheterization lab approaches, which are currently time-consuming, less accurate, effective in only about 60% of chronic cases, and associated with alarming reports of pulmonary vein stenosis and stroke. Given the high frequency of atrial fibrillation with increasing age and likely cost advantages compared to chronic medical therapy, this is an area of cardiac surgery that will likely grow over the next decades.

Transplantation

The principal limit to heart transplantation is the declining availability of donor organs. While non-heart beating donation has been developed and applied clinically for the lung and kidney, for the heart most surgeons would be uncomfortable using an organ which had stopped for any significant interval unless viability was first confirmed. Systematic assessment of organs – measuring mitochondrial reserve, oxidative state, and stress response parameters, for example, perhaps during functional evaluation in an extracorporeal circuit – might allow confident selection of good organs, particularly from older and hemodynamically unstable donors, and application of experimental interventions to restore "normal" function to organs no one will use. Resuscitation of marginal organs is probably feasible, but will require concerted application of investigative resources and careful consideration of circumstances where clinical use of such organs is ethically justified.

While it is likely to be accomplished in the near future, at present tolerance remains an elusive goal for cardiac transplant recipients. The importance of this goal is underscored by the high prevalence of cardiac allograft vasculopathy it in our patients and our inability to prevent it even with intensive suppression of the immune system. Strictly defined, tolerance is preserved function of an allograft from an unrelated individual in the absence of ongoing immune suppression; in most models it is an active "immunomodulatory" process. To achieve it, the current array of broad-spectrum immunosuppressant drugs will likely be displaced by agents that specifically interfere with pathogenic pathways, and allow emergence of active immune responses which specifically protect the graft. There has been an explosion of interest in the field, and new reagents are becoming available which selectively block individual costimulation pathways or chemokine-driven trafficking of leukocytes. However we do not yet know how to use these agents to induce tolerance, or to tell which of our patients have achieved this state. Various investigators are trying to develop tools which accurately measure whether tolerance exists, and if not, to begin to understand why.

Like tolerance, cardiac xenotransplantation is surely coming, and will likely utilize organs from pigs genetically modified ("transgenic") to express protective human genes, and deficient in proteins and sugars to which a humans mount particularly virulent responses. The only question is when the field will demonstrate sufficient progress in preclinical models to justify clinical trials, and how many modifications to the pig genome will be required to reach this point. Current approaches are likely to protect the graft from injury by complement, and to dodge the principle assault by preformed "natural" antibody. Strategies for controlling the subsequent immune response will evolve based on increased understanding of the mechanisms which drive "delayed xenograft rejection". The potential for transmission of pathogens to individual human organ recipients or dissemination into the population has been studied extensively, and the risks appear to be very small.

Long-term Mechanical Circulatory Support

Technological improvements in left ventricular assistance and artificial hearts will focus on creating safer, smaller, more energy-efficient devices. As these become available, mechanical devices will likely become "destination" therapy for many patients. Indeed, considering the side effects associated with immunosuppressive drugs, mechanical support options will likely become the definitive treatment option of choice for patients with extra cardiac pathology that would be aggravated by those drugs, and for patients who deteriorate and would otherwise die while waiting for an organ graft.

Pulsatile pumps are improving in mechanical reliability and non-pulsatile axial and centrifugal assist approaches, which are typically smaller and rely on fewer moving parts, are undergoing clinical trials. The shortcomings of many current devices in terms of infection, embolization, and mechanical failure suggest that most of them are as yet less than ideal for destination heart failure therapy. These problems should be significantly improved with the introduction of the next generation of devices. Pseudoendothelial linings associated with textured surfaces in some devices are credited with making it possible to minimize anti-coagulation, although broadly reactive alloantigen profiles in these patients raise concerns about chronic innate immune system activation. Clinical trials of completely implantable left ventricular assist and total artificial heart devices, which employ transcutaneous energy transmission, are in progress. Early results confirm that leads crossing the skin can be eliminated safely, thus removing an important source of infectious morbidity and reduced quality of life. Meanwhile rapidly improving battery technology allows patients to be untethered for significant periods of time.

In the future, incorporation of simpler connectors and improved "toolkits" as well as modular design will allow these devices to be more easily implanted, and facilitate replacement of parts in the event of device component fatigue or failure, or retrofitting of device "upgrades". A device which rapidly becomes lined by a thin layer of the patient's own endothelium would probably eliminate thrombosis and the need for intensive anticoagulation. Ongoing assessment and redesign of various pump components are likely to improve durability and reliability, and reduce thrombogenicity, creating an important growth area for future cardiac surgeons.

Gene and Cellular Therapy

Vectors for efficiently transferring genes to the endothelium or myocardium are being developed. Once the efficacy and safety of such strategies has been demonstrated, patients with ischemic heart disease may benefit from these techniques in one of several ways. Angiogenesis may recruit new blood supply to ischemic areas, while antioxidant genes might protect from additional ischemic insults. Transfection of vascular smooth muscle cells with antiproliferative molecules might prevent restenosis after stenting, or retard progression of early lesions. For future high-risk surgical candidates, preoperative transfection of cardiac myocytes with heme oxygenase, which significantly ameliorates reperfusion injury in experimental models, could be accomplished via intravascular injection at the time of diagnostic angiography. Patients suffering from heart failure may also benefit from emerging gene therapy strategies. In pre-clinical heart failure models, delivery of genes coding for proteins to regulate calcium homeostasis, beta adrenergic receptor signaling, and resistance and regulation of apoptosis have all been shown to be beneficial.

Cell transplantation may be viewed as an alternative method to genetically re-program an organ using. The description of pleuripotent mesenchymal stem cells in the heart and in other tissues has generated enthusiasm for learning how to program these cells to repair locally damaged or globally dysfunctional myocardium. In addition, our rudimentary understanding of how to control development of other pleuripotent cells from the marrow, skeletal muscle, and other tissues is expanding rapidly.

Through ex vivo exposure to as-yet-undefined patterns of growth factors, or in situ transfection with hypothetical regenerative genes, organs might be reprogrammed to repair themselves. Autologous endothelial or skeletal myoblast progenitors are particularly attractive targets for in vivo cellular transplantation after ex vivo manipulation.(7) On the other hand, reprogramming fibroblasts in areas of scar to develop synchronized contractile function seem easiest from a mechanical perspective, since they are already there, viable, and connected to each other and to the interstitial matrix.

Cardiac surgeons should look for creative ways to participate in the implementation and assessment of genetic and cell-based therapeutic approaches. It is likely that these techniques will require temporary use of cardiac assist, particularly in end-stage heart failure patients, to allow therapeutic ("reverse") ventricular remodeling under favorable hemodynamic, geometric, and biochemical conditions. Alternatively gene transfection or cell transplantation could be used in patients with early stage heart failure or coronary disease, to halt or delay progression. In either case, reliable delivery of cells and vectors with minimal systemic exposure, particularly to ischemic regions, will likely be best accomplished by direct application of genes and cells, rather than by intravascular delivery.

Culture and Education

Cardiothoracic programs have traditionally depended on general surgical training programs to deliver competent physicians and proficient technicians to them for polishing. As cardiac surgery incorporates increasingly complex technology, the duration and scope of training in this specialty will likely need to be expanded, likely coupled with expanded emphasis on teaching basic skills so as to avoid further prolongation of overall training duration. In addition, our current experience and environment suggest that the curriculum for future cardiac surgeons should include emphasis on leadership and business skills, and strategies to incorporate structured learning and quality improvement into daily clinical practice. Rapid technical evolution will generate an increasing role for the academy in career-long continuing medical education of community practitioners in cognitive and practical skills.

To avoid political impotence and favorably influencing our future work environment, our leadership is focused on aligning our interests with those of other groups. Coalitions need to be developed which include as our allies not only each other, but other physicians, the expanding community of ancillary health care providers, and – most importantly – our patients; who, after all, are voters, politicians, and opinion leaders. Where patient benefit is the focus, rather than physician income or comfort, political action on our behalf can be effectively supported to improve funding for education, quality of care, outcomes research, as well as to provide fair cardiac surgical reimbursement and promote a supportive work environment.

Summary

The next decades will continue to present us with fundamental threats, challenges to the basic assumptions around which our cardiac surgical culture and daily practice patterns are currently framed. We are required to not only achieve and document improved patient outcomes, but to do so for more difficult patients while consuming fewer resources. These complex challenges are ones for which our own training, experience, and independent practice patterns have prepared us poorly. To meet often conflicting consumer, referrer, and payer expectations, we must incorporate both evolutionary "adaptive" and revolutionary "disruptive" new technologies.(8,9) Here we have tried to touch on some of these emerging therapies and their likely impact on the cardiac surgeon's near-term future.

Culturally, rejuvenating collaborative interaction with our cardiology colleagues, and joining with them to systematically evaluate new approaches based on fair and objective outcomes assessments, seems far preferable to resorting to antagonistic attacks or direct competitive challenges. We must learn to take advantage of the fact that patients have an ever-increasing access to information about new technological advances in medicine. Naturally they will gravitate toward the newest, most advanced technology. based on the assumption that it is an improvement over time-tested "old-fashioned" approaches. However we must remain cautious about broad application of these new techniques, by us and by our cardiology colleagues, and assure that the information the patient sees is fair, objective, and complete. At present objective, unbiased assessment of new approaches is lacking, particularly at the point-of-care where critical decisions are made; and patient choices are now driven largely by provider biases and effective marketing. For example the benchmark by which other revascularization interventions must be judged remains long-term patency of mammary artery coronary bypass grafts, which confer improved patient survival.(10) Despite inferior short and long-term results, patients are easily persuaded to avoid the short-term pain and risks of major surgery in favor of catheter-based revascularization. Adapting the new technologic approaches outlined above is an obvious response, but unless we insist on incorporating benchmarks, objectively validating our new technologies, and utilizing operator-specific outcomes for continuous quality improvement, we risk compromising our current competitive advantage while jeopardizing our patients. Thus we must validate variations from standard strategies, whether based on off-pump or hybrid techniques, by careful systematic and objective follow-up.

In conclusion, we are much more likely to preserve and expand our role in managing cardiac disease if we lead the way in assessing, improving, and documenting our results, and participate actively in educating each other, our colleagues, and our patients. Taking a leadership role in safe adoption of new technology is our best strategy for diffusing the atmosphere of distrust and antagonism in which many of us now practice, and which severely impacts the psychological and emotional rewards that should attend prosecution of our remarkable therapeutic discipline.

Acknowledgment

Many of the concepts and technologies discussed here were presented in various formats at the New Era Cardiac Care Course, organized by Mehmet Oz and Randolph Chitwood, in Dana Point, CA, January 4-6, 2002; and at TechCon 2002, presented in association the annual meeting of the Society for Thoracic Surgeons, Ft. Lauderdale, FL, January 23-24, 2002. We are indebted to the many individuals who participated in these courses for both factual information and for helping us develop the conceptual framework for this chapter.

REFERENCES

1. Newman MF, Kirchner JL, Phillips-Bute B, Gaver V, Grocott H, Jones RH, Mark DB, Reves JG, Blumenthal JA. Longitudinal assessment of neurocognitive function after coronary-artery bypass surgery. N Engl J Med. 2001; 344(6): 395-402.

2. Sousa JE, Costa MA, Abizaid AC, Rensing BJ, Abizaid AS, Tanajura LF, Kozuma K, Van Langenhove G, Sousa AG, Falotico R, Jaeger J, Popma JJ, Serruys PW. Sustained suppression of neointimal proliferation by sirolimus-eluting stents: one-year angiographic and intravascular ultrasound follow-up. Circulation. 2001; 104(17): 2007-11.

3. Poon M, Badimon JJ, Fuster V. Overcoming restenosis with sirolimus: from alphabet soup to clinical reality. Lancet. 2002; 359(9306): 619-22.

4. Olinger GN. "Change in the wind": report from the 2000 Thoracic Surgery Directors Association retreat on Thoracic Surgery Graduate Medical Education. Ann Thorac Surg. 2001; 72(4): 1433-7.

5. Helman DN, Oz MC. Developing a comprehensive mechanical support program. J Card Surg. 2001; 16(3): 203-8.

6. Cox JL, Ad N, Palazzo T, Fitzpatrick S, Suyderhoud JP, DeGroot KW, Pirovic EA, Lou HC, Duvall WZ, Kim YD. Current status of the Maze procedure for the treatment of atrial fibrillation. Semin Thorac Cardiovasc Surg. 2000; 12(1): 15-9.

7. Isner, Jeffrey M., Myocardial gene therapy. Nature 2002; 415 (6868): 234-239)

8. Way LW. General surgery in evolution: technology and competence. Am J Surg. 1996; 171(1): 2-9.

9. Satava RM. Information age technologies for surgeons: overview. World J Surg. 2001; 25(11): 1408-11.

10. Lytle BW, Loop FD. Superiority of bilateral internal thoracic artery grafting: it's been a long time comin'. Circulation 2001; 104(18) :2152-4.

CHAPTER 9

ENDOCRINE SURGERY

PAUL G. GAUGER, M.D.

Introduction

"The future is no more uncertain than the present."

-Walt Whitman

The discipline of Endocrine Surgery is one of the 9 recognized principal components of General Surgery. Over the last quarter of a century, the practice of surgical endocrinology has coalesced into a distinct entity but not a separate breakaway specialty. The essence of Endocrine Surgery encompasses specific knowledge of anatomy, embryology, endocrinology, endocrine histopathology, and a background in laboratory and clinical research and experience . Endocrine Surgery deals with physiology on a molecular level, and as such, advances in recent decades have paralleled the pace and scope of changes in the "molecular age" of the medical and surgical disciplines.

Advances In Diagnostic Technology

The ability to reach a rapid and accurate preoperative diagnosis of endocrine disorders will continue to improve. Anatomic imaging for endocrine tumors is often difficult due to the small size of the tumors which may cause a profound functional or hormonal disorder without significant neoplastic "mass effects." Although it is unlikely that CT or MRI scanning will become more important for thyroid or parathyroid diseases, high-resolution ultrasound clearly will play a more prominent role. For thyroid disorders, pre-operative ultrasound performed by the operating surgeon will be used routinely to evaluate tumors and to define anatomic relationships to nerves and surrounding structures, thus assisting in surgical planning. Multiple studies suggest that ultrasound guidance lowers the rate of inadequate cytology specimens during fine needle aspiration (FNA) and may improve sensitivity and specificity. Ultrasound may be used to document normal pre-operative vocal fold mobility without patient discomfort.(2) Ultrasound will also be used by the endocrine surgeon to follow patients after resection of thyroid malignancies — both as surgeon self-appraisal in the early post-operative period and as a monitoring technique for local or regional recurrence during long-term follow up.

For parathyroid disorders, ultrasound is poised to become the preferred method of routine preoperative localization and will become even more important in providing corroborative information when ectopic cervical parathyroid adenomas are localized in patients following a failed initial exploration.(Figure 1) Some centers have developed the expertise to identify the location and size of the normal as well as abnormal parathyroid glands which will help to complete the clinicopathological picture before an operation. Intraoperative ultrasound will become more important during the parathyroidectomy procedure especially in the situation of a missing intrathyroidal parathyroid adenoma. The algorithm requiring "blind" thyroid lobectomy on the side of a missing inferior parathyroid gland will be much less rigorously followed.

Transcutaneous ultrasound is unlikely to make great strides in the evaluation of adrenal neoplasms but endoscopic ultrasound (EUS) is already the localization method of choice for pancreatic neuroendocrine neoplasms in many centers.(Figure 2) Improvement in transducer design will result in better resolution and ability to inspect the tail of the pancreas which currently is a relative blind spot. EUS will become essential in screening potentially affected family members for the pancreatic tumors associated with the Multiple Endocrine Neoplasia 1 syndrome.

Endocrine Surgery depends heavily on functional imaging to enhance anatomic imaging in many situations. Changes will continue to occur in the general areas of preoperative localization and postoperative tumor imaging. The same compounds may be used in targeted tumor therapy. Preoperative localization of parathyroid tumors often uses the technetium-based compound, Tc 99m sestamibi. As the radionuclide works by concentrating in the mitochondria of abnormal parathyroid glands, it is likely that compounds will be developed which either facilitate sestamibi entry into, or delay washout from, the mitochondria of these abnormal parathyroid cells to enhance imaging.

The range of nuclear imaging compounds will be expanded and will include antibodies and additional ligands to facilitate imaging of parathyroid and other endocrine tumors. Somatostatin receptor scintigraphy has become commonplace for endocrine tumors. The success of this modality is based on in-vitro somatostatin receptor autoradiography which has demonstrated somatostatin receptors in 100% of gastrinomas, glucagonomas, and non-functioning pancreatic endocrine tumors, and 72% of insulinomas.(3) The in-vivo clinical sensitivity is less profound, but the technique is rapidly becoming the imaging modality of choice for patients with gastrinomas, carcinoid tumors, and non-insulinoma gastroenteropancreatic neuroendocrine tumors.(Figure 3) Improved collimation and scintigraphic data reconstruction techniques will improve the spatial resolution of this technique. The sensitivity of such studies will be improved by development of ligand compounds for additional somatostatin receptor subtypes. Perhaps, entirely new radionuclides will exploit novel receptors not yet discovered.

Management of the follicular thyroid neoplasm continues to vex endocrine surgeons and is still a deficiency in optimal patient management. Surgeons will soon

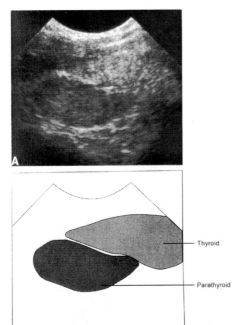

Figure 9-1

Sonographic detection of a large parathyroid adenoma. Reproduced with permission from Ultrasound in Surgical Practice: Basic Principles and Clinical Applications. JK Harness and DB Wisher, eds. John Wiley & Sons, Inc., New York NY. 2002.

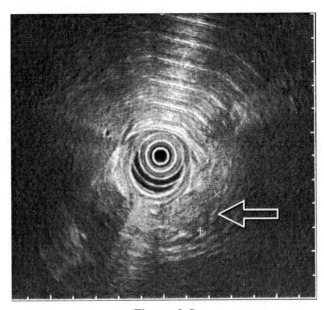

Figure 9-2

Endoscopic ultrasound (EUS) delineating a solitary insulinoma in within the substance of the pancreas.

have available markers which will discriminate follicular carcinoma from follicular adenomas and thus allow more appropriate patient selection for surgery. One such marker may be PAX8-PPARg1, a fusion oncoprotein present in follicular carcinomas but not follicular adenomas or papillary carcinomas.(4) Fine needle aspiration specimens will eventually be submitted to an analysis panel of oncogenes and operations for benign follicular adenomas will greatly decrease.

The genetic mutations leading to the recognized syndromes of Multiple Endocrine Neoplasia (MEN 1, MEN 2A, MEN 2B) have now been well characterized and additional familial syndromes will continue to be defined. The clinical definition of MEN 1 has been expanded to include other associated conditions such as carcinoid, thyroid, and adrenocortical tumors. This new understanding will increase the recognition of the syndrome and lead to increased use of genetic analysis for diagnostic confirmation and analysis of the patient's kindred. The number and location of mutations in MEN 1 leading to the production of a dysfunctional protein product (menin) are already multitudinous but will continue to expand. Various genotype / phenotype correlations will be defined which will influence clinical screening for specific lesions. As medicine and society at large increase their "comfort level" with genetic screening, many laboratories will routinely offer such studies. RET proto-oncogene analysis will continue to be an integral part of the management of the patient and the family in MEN 2A and 2B as well as familial medullary thyroid cancer. In similar fashion to MEN 1, the number of defined codon mutations associated with MEN 2 will be expanded. As genetic analysis plays an enhanced role in management of en-

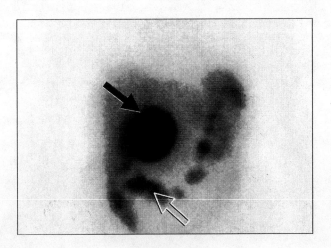

Figure 9-3
Somatostatin Receptor Scintigraphy (Octreotide Scanning) in a patient with an exceptionally large neuroendocrine tumor of the head of the pancreas.

docrine neoplasms, the requirement for expert genetic counselors will grow and such a program will be an integral part of any tertiary care setting. Endocrine surgeons have already established many such programs around the world.

Advances In Procedural And Therapeutic Technology

The last decade has witnessed a proliferation of technological enhancements in surgery leading to minimally invasive alternative procedures in many areas of General Surgery. As expected, these changes have occurred in Endocrine Surgery as well. These techniques are often optimally suited for endocrine patients as many of the tumors removed are small, benign, and difficult to expose with standard surgical techniques. It is all too easy to look toward the future and predict that soon, nearly all operations will be done in a minimally invasive, endoscopic, laparoscopic, or even robot-assisted fashion. It is more likely, however, that these advanced techniques will not eliminate standard surgical techniques. Lessons learned from advances in technique will add new emphasis to proper patient selection. The costs of increased material and time which are generated by technology-based approaches will need to be justified in the domain of cost effectiveness.

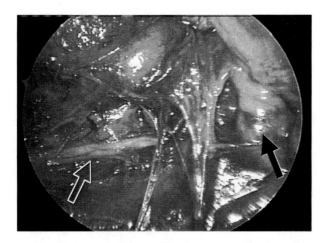

Figure 9-4
Video image from an endoscopic thyroidectomy for a solitary thyroid nodule. Note the recurrent laryngeal nerve (white outlined arrow) and the superior parathyroid gland (black arrow). Image acquired and provided by William B. Inabnet, M.D.

A good example of this equipoise is found in the area of thyroid surgery. Investigators in many countries have described the advantages of endoscopic thyroid resections.(Figure 4) Access is variably provided through cervical ports or even subcutaneous chest wall or axillary ports. The premise guiding these alternatives is that conventional neck surgery is cosmetically and functionally disabling to the patient. This assertion is not well documented and it will be difficult for expensive, technology-laden alternatives such as these to surpass the safety and efficacy of the conventional thyroid resection. The procedures will continue to be performed as long as patients seek these alternatives but have yet to be accepted as the new standard of care.

Parathyroid surgery has already undergone a revolution, or perhaps an evolution, to limit the scope of the operation. This will be a lasting change. The standard of care has long been mandatory operative identification of all 4 parathyroid glands without preoperative localization. This standard has already changed due to factors such as improved preoperative localization by ultrasound or by sestamibi SPECT scanning. Another factor catalyzing change has been the emergence of intraoperative parathyroid hormone monitoring. Unfortunately, neither preoperative localization nor intraoperative parathyroid hormone monitoring is perfect at detecting multiglandular disease which continues to be the Achilles' heel of the surgical treatment of hyperparathyroidism. The combination of the "health-care consumer" role of the modern patient and the market forces provided by the Internet proved to be a major driving impetus for the operation to evolve to a more concise version. Limiting the scope of the operation may make parathyroidectomy more "accessible" to the less experienced surgeon and this may negatively impact the overall success rate of surgical intervention. However, because of the limited scope of the initial operation, the character of subsequent reoperation for patients with persistent or recurrent hyperparathyroidism may also be less complicated. As an effect of these many factors, the gold standard paradigm for parathyroidectomy will soon shift to a targeted operation which depends on preoperative localization and intraoperative hormone monitoring with the possible result that the long term cure rate of the initial operation will decrease slightly. In some sense, this can be viewed as a compromise in principles and the acceptability of these changes will continue to be debated in the Endocrine Surgical community.

Laparoscopic adrenalectomy has become the preferred approach for benign surgical diseases of the adrenal gland and the advantages over laparotomy are clear. As is the case with many laparoscopic procedures, the technique has sometimes been applied inappropriately. Patients with adrenocortical carcinoma resected by a laparoscopic approach often have rapid and unresectable local recurrences of their cancer within the adrenal bed. Laparoscopic adrenalectomy has already been accepted as the new standard approach for benign adrenal lesions. Even so, laparoscopic adrenalectomy may never gain the widespread acceptance of laparoscopic cholecystectomy because of 2 principal factors: the increased technical difficulty compared with cholecystectomy and the small number of patients requiring adrenalectomy.(5) The retroperitoneal posterior approach will become more common as an alternative to the transperitoneal flank approach.

Pancreatic endocrine tumors are often histologically benign and have a benign clinical course even if a locally infiltrative tumor can be resected completely. Experience is increasing with laparoscopic enucleation or resection of tumors such as insulinomas. This approach will likely become the standard as improved preoperative imaging allows optimum patient selection. The selection of patients with benign disease is based on the tumor's relationship to surrounding normal tissue and the presence or absence of enlarged surrounding lymph nodes. Laparoscopic ultrasound will also have an increased role in these operations. The technically precise act of enucleation may be optimally performed via a laparoscopic approach with robotic assistance — especially for lesions in the pancreatic body and tail. This option may be less applicable for tumors in the head of the pancreas where intraoperative palpation is a relatively more important method of localization. Perhaps these pancreatic head lesions will benefit from hybrid approaches such as hand-assisted laparoscopic surgery.

Just as the diagnostic aspects of Endocrine Surgery have come to rely heavily on radionuclide functional imaging, this approach has already been carried into the operating room. Radioguided surgery has been one of the heavily promoted aspects of minimally invasive parathyroid surgery that has driven the evolution of that operation. Neither the radionuclide used (sestamibi) nor the hand-held gamma detector is perfectly suited for this application and may not materially change the sequence or success of the operation.(6) The spatial resolution of the probe itself will be improved and perhaps a compound that prolongs sestamibi retention in abnormal parathyroid glands or promotes washout in other non-parathyroid tissues will improve the sensitivity of this technique. The spectrum of radioguided surgery will also expand by exploiting somatostatin receptors present in many neuroendocrine tumors. Intraoperative radioguidance is already being used for carcinoid tumors and it follows that it may soon be an important aspect of surgery for gastrinomas or other pancreatic endocrine tumors. Less certain is the role of radioguidance in patients with malignant pheochromocytoma. Investigators have begun work on a probe capable of detecting 18F-Fluorodeoxyglucose activity intraoperatively, thus widening the potential applications of this compound in patients with positive PET scans.(7)

Intraoperative hormone monitoring has become common as an adjunct to parathyroid operations and the very nature of endocrine surgery points to many other future directions for this exciting technology. Intraoperative hormone monitoring has evolved from standard assay techniques to rapid chemiluminescent assays. To be useful and cost- or time-effective, hormone assays should provide feedback in less than 15 - 20 minutes.

The limits of intraoperative parathyroid hormone monitoring are still being defined and this technique has caused surgeons to reevaluate the definition of multiglandular parathyroid disease. Increased parathyroid gland size is not necessarily synonymous with hyperfunction.(8) Even so, intraoperative parathyroid hormone monitoring will become a standard and necessary adjunct to any targeted, or minimally invasive, parathyroidectomy.

There is a similar need for intraoperative monitoring of gastrin levels to assess complete resection of gastrinoma. The concept has been validated using standard gastrin assays but a practical rapid assay is not yet available.(9) This is purely a technical limitation of the assay and it will be overcome. Intraoperative gastrin monitoring will become a standard adjunct to operation for sporadic and familial gastrinoma.

After resection of an insulinoma, intraoperative blood glucose levels should rise when the tumor has been completely removed but this is a rather gross indication of success. Rapid insulin assays are in use in Japan but are not yet widely available. Again, this is an issue which will be overcome by improved assay techniques and measurement of insulin, or perhaps proinsulin, will be routine during operation for insulinoma.

As medicine has evolved to a molecular approach for understanding and treating diseases, patients with endocrine tumors stand to profit disproportionally as many of the diseases are clearly mediated by molecular markers and signaling processes. The availability and use of somatostatin analogues such as octreotide acetate has substantially changed the treatment of some patients with neuroendocrine tumors. In many cases, this compound is able to improve control of hormonally mediated symptoms and thus improve patient quality of life. Data are incomplete, but the hormone may even act as a tumor-static agent in some patients with metastatic gastroenteropancreatic neuroendocrine tumors. A long acting depot preparation is now available and its use will become common. OctreoTher™ is a radionuclide which may hold promise in targeting and treating tumors with somatostatin subtype 2 receptors and this agent will undergo substantial further evaluation.

Surgery has been standard therapy for primary hyperparathyroidism and medical management has largely consisted of observation or therapy aimed at reducing end-organ complications such as osteoporosis. This may change as drugs become available to address the physiologic perturbations of hyperparathyroidism. One such drug is the calcium receptor antagonist R-568 which has already shown temporary efficacy.(10) Endocrine surgeons should be proactive patient advocates in this area and are optimally poised to lead well-conducted prospective, randomized trials comparing such short and long term medical therapy with surgical cure.

Poorly differentiated thyroid malignancies will be treated by novel approaches such as "redifferentiation" therapy. This has already been accomplished by treatment of 131I refractory thyroid cancers with 13-cis-retinoic acid which may renew radioiodine uptake in some patients.(11) Poorly differentiated thyroid carcinomas are often deficient in the sodium iodide symporter and this is responsible for their inability to take up radioiodine. A very exciting direction for the future is to target gene therapy at reconstituting this function again allowing radioiodine use for treatment.(12)

The most uniformly fatal endocrine neoplasm remains anaplastic thyroid cancer. Some isolated anaplastic thyroid cancers express multidrug resistance associated proteins. Approaches to inactivate these proteins will result in more efficacious chemotherapy which will more commonly utilize paclitaxel. The compound ST1571 (Gleevec) has a potential future role in treatment of some thyroid malignancies such as medullary thyroid carcinoma by virtue of its RET tyrosine kinase activity and perhaps even anaplastic thyroid cancer via interaction with platelet derived growth factor.

Advances In The Discipline Of Endocrine Surgery

The International Association of Endocrine Surgeons was established in 1979 and the American Association of Endocrine Surgeons was founded just one year later, holding its first meeting in Ann Arbor, Michigan. Both societies have continued to grow and thrive.

Endocrine operative procedures will become more concentrated in academic health centers or specialty clinics. This will occur for a number of reasons including the development and evaluation of novel therapies and procedures by research based institutions. Perhaps even more influential will be the public dissemination of outcomes and complication data which will tend to reflect favorably on academic centers. This is already occurring in a consumer-driven fashion but academic centers will soon join in this effort. Cost effectiveness and superior outcome and complication data will also dictate referral patterns for patients under many different insurance carriers. A more formalized undergraduate, graduate, and post-graduate educational structure for the future practitioners of endocrine surgery will also tend to be more common in academic centers.

To deserve this vital and exciting practice environment, academic centers must become leaders in interdisciplinary care. With lessons learned from breast care, Endocrine Surgery will evolve to a "Center of Excellence" approach.(13) Surgeons will need to foster even better relationships with our endocrinology, pathology, radiology, and nuclear medicine colleagues to streamline and optimize optimal patient care.

Improved studies of patient outcomes will influence the prevalence of some endocrine procedures and relegate others to the realm of medical history. The best efforts so far in outcomes based endocrine surgery research have taken place in the area of parathyroid surgery and have already led to increased referrals for these procedures.(14, 15) The influences of volume and expertise on cure and complications have also been evaluated in the context of regional health care delivery and these sorts of outcomes documentation will further promote the concentration of endocrine procedures in academic centers.(16, 17)

Clinical research will be greatly enhanced by innovative database designs which will facilitate complex queries interrelating clinical, genetic, pathologic, and financial data. The potential here is profound, but success is not guaranteed as societal forces increasingly limit how these data can be collected, stored, and accessed.

One of the factors driving the future concentration of endocrine operations in tertiary centers will be the burgeoning literature on cost-effectiveness. The cost of a failed initial parathyroidectomy has already been documented and avoiding initial failure by providing expert care will both save health care dollars and protect the patient.(18) This issue will be central if minimally invasive parathyroidectomy techniques ultimately meet with a slightly lessened long-term success rate. However, it may be argued that the abbreviated parathyroidectomy of the future will also be more cost effective in the short term based on decreased operative time and outpatient treatment but only if adjunctive technologies are used with discrimination. The obvious intersection of these two issues is the question of long term cost effectiveness of the targeted parathyroidectomy if the durable cure rate is eroded and more patients ultimately require reoperation.

Ever since the recognition of Endocrine Surgery as a separate subspecialty aspect of General Surgery, a great deal of attention has been paid to defining adequate experience and training. A recent survey of graduating medical students beginning a career in surgery revealed that 34% failed to see a single thyroid operation, 42% failed to see any parathyroid operation, and 65% failed to see an adrenalectomy during their surgical rotations.(19) Even more concerning is the fact that practical clinical experience during a General Surgery residency can also be quite limited. This deficiency is related to the low natural incidence of endocrine diseases requiring operation and may also be related to the incursion of other competing surgical specialties or factors such as the lack of dedicated endocrine surgeon on the teaching faculty. For programs without an identified endocrine surgeon in 1995, the mean numbers of procedures performed as a resident were only 12.5 ± 6.1 thyroid operations, 4.9 ± 2.5 parathyroid operations, 1.3 ± 0.8 adrenal operations, and 0.2 ± 0.4 endocrine pancreatic operations.(20) Leaders in the field have suggested that it is in the best interest of future patients and of the specialty itself to institute a formalized curriculum and system for advanced training in endocrine surgery — lasting as long as 2 additional years.(20, 21) This is likely to occur in tertiary centers where this educational mission can be subsidized. However, it is unlikely the there will be a separate board examination beyond a certificate of special qualification in endocrine surgery.(22)

Conclusion

Secretin was the first hormone to be described over a century ago. The name of the hormone was derived from Latin meaning "something secret" or "a mystery." The term hormone was derived from the Greek "to excite." Indeed, the future of Endocrine Surgery promises to have an ample supply of both mystery and excitement. The next twenty years will bring fascinating advancements in diagnostic and treatment modalities in Endocrine Surgery as well as changes in the definition and vitality of the field itself.

REFERENCES

1. Paloyan E. American Association of Endocrine Surgeons presidential address: The Gatekeepers. Surgery 1988;104:937-939.

2. Hsiao TY, Wang CL, Chen CN, Hsieh FJ, Shau YW. Noninvasive assessment of laryngeal phonation function using color Doppler ultrasound imaging. Ultrasound in Medicine & Biology 2001;27:1035-1040.

3. Krenning EP, Kwekkeboom DJ, Reubi JC, vanHagen PM, vanEijck CH, Oei HY, et al. 111In-ocreotide scintigraphy in oncology. Digestion 1993;54 (suppl):84-87.

4. Kroll TG, Sarraf P, Pecciarini L, Chen CJ, Mueller E, Spiegelman BM, et al. PAX8-PPARg1 fusion oncogen in human thyroid carcinoma. Science 2000;289:1357-1360.

5. van Heerden JA. What's new in endocrine surgery? Journal of the American College of Surgeons 1998;186:141-148.

6. Dackiw APB, Sussman JJ, Fritsche HA, Delpassand ES, Stanford P, Hoff A, et al. Relative contributions of technetium Tc 99m sestamibi scintigraphy, intraoperative gamma probe detection, and the rapid parathyroid hormone assay to the surgical management of hyperparathyroidism. Archives of Surgery 2000;135:550-557.

7. Yasuda S, Makuuchi H, Fujii H, Nakasaki H, Mukai M, Sadahiro S, et al. Evaluation of a surgical gamma probe for detection of 18F-FDG. Tokai Journal of Experimental & Clinical Medicine 2000;25:93-99.

8. Gauger PG, Agarwal G, England BG, Delbridge LW, Matz KA, Wilkinson M, et al. Intraoperative parathyroid hormone monitoring fails to detect double parathyroid adenomas: A 2-institution experience. Surgery 2001;130:1005-1010.

9. Proye C, Pattou F, Carnaille B, Paris JC, d'Herbomez M, Marchandise X. Intraoperative gastrin measurements during surgical management of patients with gastrinomas: experience with 20 cases. World Journal of Surgery 1998;22:643-649.

10. Silverberg SJ, 3rd HGB, Marriott TB, Locker FG, Thys-Jacobs S, Dziem G, et al. Short-term inhibition of parathyroid hormone secretion by a calcium-receptor agonist in patients with primary hyperparathyroidism. New England Journal of Medicine 1997;337:1506-1510.

11. Simon D, Kohrle J, Schmutzler C, Mainz K, Reiners C, Roher HD. Redifferentiation therapy of differentiated thyroid carcinoma with retinoic acid: basics and first clinical results. Experimental & Clinical Endocrinology & Diabetes 1996;104 (Suppl 4):13-15.

12. Smit JW, Shroder-van der Elst JP, Karperien M, Que I, van der Pluijm G, Goslings B, et al. Reestablishment of in vitro and in vivo iodide uptake by transfection of the human sodium iodide symporter (hNIS) in a hNIS defective human thyroid carcinoma cell line. Thyroid 2000;10:939-943.

13. Harness JK. American Association of Endocrine Surgeons presidential address: Interdisciplinary care-the future of endocrine surgery. Surgery 2000;128:873-880.

14. Burney RE, Jones KR, Christy B, Thompson NW. Health status improvement after surgical correction of primary hyperparathyroidism in patients with high and low preoperative calcium levels. Surgery 1999;125:608-614.

15. Solomon BL, Schaaf M, Smallridge RC. Psychologic symptoms before and after parathyroid surgery. American Journal of Medicine 1994;96:101-106.

16. Sosa JA, Bowman HM, Tielsch JM, Powe NR, Gordon TA, Udelsman R. The importance of surgeon experience for clinical and economic outcomes from thyroidectomy. Annals of Surgery 1998;228:320-330.

17. Chen H, Zeiger MA, Gordon TA, Udelsman R. Parathyroidectomy in Maryland: effects of an endocrine center. Surgery 1996;120:948-958.

18. Doherty GM, Weber B, Norton JA. Cost of unsuccessful surgery for primary hyperparathyroidism. Surgery 1994;116:954-958.

19. Chen HC, Hardacre JM, Martin C, Udelsman R, Lillemoe KD. Do future general surgery residents have adequate exposure to endocrine surgery during medical school? World Journal of Surgery 2002;26:17-21.

20. Prinz RA. American Association of Endocrine Surgeons presidential address: Endocrine surgical training-some ABC measures. Surgery 1996;120:905-912.

21. Harness JK, van Heerden JA, Lennquist S, Rothmund M, Barraclough BH, Goode AW, et al. Future of thyroid surgery and training surgeons to meet the expectations of 2000 and beyond. World Journal of Surgery 2000;24:976-982.

22. Thompson NW. The evolution of endocrine surgery as a subspecialty of general surgery. Fragmentation or enhancement? Archives of Surgery 1996;131:465-471.

CHAPTER 10

GASTROINTESTINAL SURGERY

LISA COLLETTI, M.D.

Introduction

The advances in medicine and surgery that have occurred over the past 50 years have been astounding. The practice of surgery today would have been unimaginable to a practitioner 50 years ago. Who would have predicted that gallbladders could be removed almost painlessly using four less than 2 centimeter incisions and that the vast majority of patients would undergo this procedure on an outpatient basis? Advances in medical technology have been amazing and the changes in this area are now progressing at an exponential rate. The changes in the next 50 years will likely far outstrip those of the past 50 years.

The Patient

People are living longer and often enjoy a good quality of life in advanced years. The average life expectancy for a man in 1900 was 46 years, and for a woman 49 years; currently, the average life span for a man is 72 years, and for a woman 79 years.(1) The geriatric population, those individuals over the age of 65, currently composes 13% of the US population, but encompass 37% of discharges from acute care hospitals in this country.(2) Continued improvement in the quality of life for the increasing geriatric patient population, along with the increases in overall life span, should be the goal for the medical community. Surgeons need to be aware of the special needs of the geriatric patient and the physiologic changes that occur as people age, particularly as the geriatric population in the United States continues to grow.

The result of aging is not disease, but decreased physiologic reserve. Because of decrease in physiologic reserve, disease can present at an early stage in the elderly, with symptoms commonly developing in the weakest organ system. Immune function declines with age; thus, the inflammatory response to an acute insult may be blunted, causing the elderly patient to present with more subtle or somewhat different signs in the setting of an acute surgical problem, resulting in a delay in diagnosis. Some physiologic changes that occur during the process of aging include a decrease in vital capacity, a decrease in immune function, a decrease in bronchociliary movement, and an increase in arterial wall stiffness. Overall aerobic capacity also declines.

A recent investigation has demonstrated that when an elderly patient is hospitalized for an acute medical illness, hospitalization is often followed by progressive deterioration, with a high mortality rate during the first year following discharge.(3) Six independent risk factors have been defined which predict mortality for elderly patients in this setting.(3) These risk factors are outlined in Table 1.

Over 50% of the cancer incidence and 67% of the cancer mortality occurs in patients greater than age 65 of age.(4) These disproportionate statistics will likely increase over the next decades, with an aging population. The elderly patient presents special challenges for any planned operative intervention, but particularly when major operative procedures for gastrointestinal malignancies are anticipated. Some of these include diagnostic delays, increased procedure-related risks due to concurrent comorbid conditions, and special support needs. Overall survival is generally shorter. Several recent studies suggest that the geriatric patient is not at increased risk for a poor outcome or more frequent or severe complications after major abdominal operations, even in the setting of malignancy.(5,6) Mortality and length of stay were not significantly different in older patient groups in these studies; advanced age did, however, predict an increased risk of some post-operative complications, such as hemorrhage and relaparotomy.(5,6) Given other investigations documenting improved survival following major cancer operations in centers which do a high volume of these procedures, it will likely be important in the future to concentrate these types of procedures in high volume centers, especially for the geriatric patient.(7)

Diagnostic Techniques And Imaging
Computed Tomographic Scanning (CT Scanning)

Helical, or spiral, CT scanning has significantly improved CT-generated images, and has also allowed for the development of more sophisticated examinations using this technology, such as CT angiography. Advanced 3-D processing is the basis for even more sophisticated imagery, such as virtual colonoscopy. This technology now enables the radiologist to view anatomy from within any lumen or anatomic space within the body.

Table 1. Risk factors for 1 year mortality following hospitalization for an acute medical illness in elderly patients (53).

Male gender

Number of dependent activities of daily living at discharge

Congestive heart failure

Cancer

Creatinine >3 mg/dl

Low albumin <3.0 g/dl

Hepatic Imaging

Helical CT scanning represents a significant improvement in hepatic imaging over standard CT scanning.(Table 2) The relatively short scan time allows the entire liver to be imaged during the time of peak tissue contrast enhancement, without scanning during the equilibrium phase, allowing optimal tissue visualization.(8) The liver can also be imaged during the arterial and/or portal venous phases of contrast enhancement (dual phase scanning), facilitating optimal visualization of certain types of neoplasms.(8) For example, colorectal metastases are typically hypovascular compared to normal hepatic parenchyma and are imaged optimally during the portal venous phase.(8) Many primary hepatic neoplasms, such as hepatocellular carcinoma, are hypervascular, and are optimally visualized during the hepatic arterial phase.(8) The overall resolution of this type of scanning is also superior and allows detection of smaller lesions.

Table 2. Advantages of Helical CT Scanning

Speed of scanning

Imaging at peak tissue levels of contrast material

Need for decreased doses of contrast material

Decrease/obliteration of respiratory variation

Ability to image arterial and venous systems

Ability to perform 3-D reconstructions to provide additional information

---

Pancreatic Imaging

Helical CT is provides excellent, high resolution imaging of the pancreas. In addition to detecting relatively small lesions, as compared to standard CT scanning, helical CT is also very sensitive for the detection of portal vein, superior mesenteric vein and/or superior mesenteric artery involvement by pancreatic neoplasms.(8) All of the splanchnic arteries and veins may be evaluated with a dedicated spiral CT angiogram. These vessels may also be retrospectively evaluated with post-processing techniques applied to previously obtained routine abdominal spiral CT's. Helical CT imaging or spiral CT angiography may be used to specifically evaluate the hepatic artery and portal vein, in order to define hepatic arterial anatomy and to detect hepatic arterial or portal venous thrombosis. This technique can be used as part of the preoperative evaluation of patients who are candidates for hepatic resection or liver transplantation.(8)

Magnetic Resonance Imaging (MRI)

Standard MRI is most useful in the area of gastrointestinal (GI) surgery for hepatic imaging. Two new liver imaging contrast agents, ferumoxide and mangafodipir trisodium, have increased the sensitivity of MRI for the detection and characterization of hepatic lesions.(9)

Manganese-enhanced MRI is also beneficial for pancreatic imaging, although fat-suppressed, T1-weighted imaging with gadolinium enhancement yields results which are comparable to helical CT scanning.(9) Magnetic resonance (MR) vascular imaging, particularly portal venography, is useful in the evaluation of the Budd-Chiari syndrome and for evaluating for portal venous invasion in patients with pancreatic cancer.(9)

The development of phased-array body coils and endorectal coils produce high quality MR images of perirectal disease, including that associated with Crohn's disease, complex fistula-in-ano, and in post-partum sphincter dysfunction.(9) As MR techniques continue to evolve, MR virtual endoscopy will also become feasible. Magnetic resonance enteroscopy allows complete visualization of the entire GI tract and may eventually make endoscopy obsolete for diagnostic interventions, relegating endoscopic techniques solely to therapeutic interventions.(10)

Magnetic Resonance Cholangiopancreatography (MRCP)

This relatively new technique is a non-invasive method for the evaluation of patients with pancreaticobiliary disease. MRCP produces comparable results and images to the more invasive technique of endoscopic retrograde cholangiopancreatography (ERCP) for the diagnosis of extrahepatic biliary abnormalities, including stones and benign and malignant strictures.(Table 3) MRCP has a further advantage over ERCP in that it provides additional data regarding the extent of disease, specifically information regarding the presence of distant metastatic disease, and possibly by demonstrating the presence of enlarged lymph nodes. MRCP is clearly the imaging modality of choice for patients with biliary-enteric anastomoses, which preclude

---

Table 3. Limitations to MRCP

> Patient motion or inability to breath-hold
>
> Patient irregular respirations
>
> Severe pneumobilia
>
> Severe ascites
>
> Presence of metal implants in the patient's body
>
> Patient claustrophobia

access to the pancreaticobiliary tree by ERCP. MRCP is also a relatively sensitive technique for the detection of pancreas divisum.(11) Since MRCP is increasingly utilized for diagnosis, the emphasis on ERCP will shift from diagnostic to therapeutic. For predicting resectability in the preoperative evaluation of pancreatic masses, MRI combined with MRCP resulted in a 100% sensitivity, 83% specificity, a positive predictive value of 94%, a negative predictive value of 100%, and an accuracy of 95%.(12)

Fluorodeoxyglucose Positron Emission Tomography (FDG PET)

The unique biology of cancer cells allows the functional imaging performed by PET scanning to differentiate benign from malignant lesions. FDG-PET is a sensitive diagnostic tool that images tumors based on increased uptake of glucose by tumor cells; in general, tumor cells are metabolically more active than normal cells in the same vicinity. FDG is transported through the GLUT glucose transporter, is phosphorylated by hexokinase, and metabolically trapped.

Several recent studies have documented the successful use of this modality for evaluation of GI tract malignancies. In patients with pancreatic masses, PET is useful in differentiating pancreatic carcinoma from chronic focal pancreatitis.(13) PET is also useful for evaluation of both primary and metastatic hepatic lesions. In relatively large study evaluating 110 patients with new hepatic lesions, PET was 100% accurate in all patients with liver metastases from adenocarcinoma and sarcoma primaries.(14) A small percentage of false positive results were noted in patients with hepatic abscesses and a small number of false negative results were seen in patients with hepatocellular carcinoma.(14) This technique was also useful in monitoring response to therapy and for detection of recurrence, both intra- and extra-hepatic.(14) FDG PET is particularly accurate and sensitive for the detection of hepatic and extra-hepatic colorectal metastases, and when used in conjunction with other imaging modalities often alters patient management due to the detection of additional metastatic disease. In one study of patients with metastatic colorectal cancer being referred for hepatic resection of their metastases, PET imaging detected additional metastatic disease in approximately 25% of the patients studied.(15) A large meta-analysis of the literature suggests that PET has a 97% sensitivity, 75% specificity, and changes patient management in 29% of patients with recurrent colorectal cancer.(16)

Endoscopic Ultrasounds (EUS)

Endoscopic ultrasonography allows endoscopic imaging of lesions within and beyond the lumen of the gastrointestinal tract. This technology enables endoscopists to image and biopsy mural, transmural, paraluminal, mediastinal, pelvic, and retroperitoneal pathology.(17) For the gastrointestinal surgeon, this technique has the

Table 4. Indications for EUS (15)

Upper GI Tract

Staging of malignancies of the esophagus, stomach, and possibly duodenum

Diagnosis of submucosal lesions, differentiation of benign and malignant stromal tumors

Evaluation of anastomotic strictures (esophageal and rectal)

Pancreatico-biliary system

Staging/evaluation of pancreatic masses

Staging/evaluation of ampullary masses

Diagnosis of CBD stones

Possible differential diagnosis of chronic pancreatitis

Anorectal Area

Staging of rectal cancer

Evaluation of the anal sphincter

Other applications

Ability to perform fine needle aspiration of masses in and around the GI tract

Celiac neurolysis for pain control in patients with unresectable pancreatic cancer.

---

greatest application toward imaging of pancreatic head lesions, esophageal and gastric lesions, and rectal lesions, as well as differentiating benign and malignant GI stromal tumors.(Table 4) (17-22)

EUS and Pancreatic Lesions

For pancreatic head lesions, in addition to being able to sample the tumor for diagnostic purposes, EUS also allows accurate analysis of tumor involvement of the superior mesenteric and portal veins, and the superior mesenteric artery.(17, 22) Lymph nodes in the region of the tumor can also be imaged with this technology. In a meta-analysis of the current literature, EUS was 98% sensitive for diagnosing pancreatic cancer (18) and was superior to all other imaging modalities, including standard ultrasonography (75%), CT (80%), and angiography (89%). Although the EUS sensitivity rates are high, the specificity rates have been lower due to difficulty in differentiating focal chronic pancreatitis from cancer. Both of these lesions can appear as focal hypoechoic areas within the substance of the pancreas. When other findings suggesting more advanced disease are appreciated, such as vessel invasion, lymphadenopathy, and pancreatic ductal obstruction, the diagnostic accuracy of EUS is increased and approaches 80%; when combined with EUS-guided biopsy, the specificity increases to 88%.(23) EUS is also useful for TNM staging of pancreatic tumors, and in a compilation of a large number of studies involving a total of 350 patients, EUS was 80% accurate for T staging, and 72% accurate for detection of nodal metastases.(24) EUS was found to be equivalent to angiography for the detection of portal venous invasion (85% vs 83%) (25) and was also equivalent to helical CT scanning for overall local staging of pancreatic malignancies (approximately 93%).(26) EUS does have the disadvantage of not being able to detect distant metastatic disease, as compared to CT scanning. EUS is also useful for the diagnosis of other pancreatic disorders, including chronic pancreatitis, cystic neoplasms of the pancreas, and neuroendocrine tumors of the pancreas.

A recent therapeutic advance in EUS allows EUS-guided celiac nerve block. Recent data suggests that this technique is safe and provides effective, long-lasting pain relief for the majority of patients with pain related to upper abdominal GI malignancies, most commonly pancreatic cancer.(21) In a single treatment setting, EUS can provide accurate diagnosis, staging, and palliation of pain for patients with unresectable pancreatic cancer.

EUS and Luminal Malignancies

EUS is very useful for staging of esophageal, gastric and rectal malignancies.(17,20,22) EUS visualizes the distinct histologic layers of the esophageal, gastric and rectal walls, in addition to imaging lymph nodes in the vicinity.(17,20,22) This technique can determine if esophageal, gastric or rectal tumors are localized to the mucosa-submucosa (T1-T2 lesions) or have invaded through the muscularis propria (T3); EUS can also document invasion of extraintestinal structures, corresponding to T4 lesions.

This technique is more useful for the staging of esophageal tumors. Many studies have documented an accuracy of EUS-based TN staging the range of 70-90% for esophageal malignancies.(22) The accuracy of EUS for T staging of esophageal carcinoma is 80-90%, and is significantly greater than that reported for CT scanning, which ranges from 50-60%. EUS-based nodal staging for esophageal cancers is not quite as accurate as T staging, but still averages approximately 75%, and is still substantially higher than that for CT scanning (54%) (27), although CT scanning still has an important role for the documentation of distant metastatic disease. When EUS is combined with CT scanning, the diagnostic accuracy for the staging of esophageal carcinoma is approximately 86% (27); accuracy of staging in this disease process is important as it has a significant impact on treatment selection. EUS is also very accurate for detecting esophageal anastomotic recurrence, with accuracy rates ranging 80% (28); this accuracy is increased if combined with fine needle aspiration (FNA).

EUS-based staging of gastric carcinoma uses the same principles as associated with esophageal cancer, but has been less well-studied than esophageal staging.(22) One of the major limitations of EUS is its inability to differentiate between benign peritumoral edema and malignant infiltration. The presence of edema is the most common source for inaccurate staging, particularly for gastric lesions.(22) This is particularly problematic when attempting to use EUS to differentiate between a benign and malignant gastric ulcer.(22) A number of criteria have been developed to differentiate benign and malignant stromal tumors, but they have not yet been rigorously tested. Irregular, heterogenous masses with a diameter of >4 cm should be considered to be suspicious for malignancy.(19)

EUS is also highly useful for the TNM staging of rectal cancers, and has an accuracy of 73-94% when performed prior to radiation therapy.(29) As discussed above, one of the major limitations of EUS is its inability to differentiate between benign peritumoral edema and malignant infiltration, and the use of EUS following radiation therapy is compromised by the development of peritumoral edema associated with treatment.

Gastrointestinal Endoscopy
Esophagogastroduodenoscopy

Progress in gastrointestinal endoscopic technology parallels that seen with laparoscopic technology and robotics. The development of ultrathin endoscopes may permit sedationless endoscopy. The standard gastroscope diameter is currently 9-11 mm, corresponding to diagnostic and therapeutic endoscopes. The newer ultrathin endoscopes have an outer diameter of 5.3-5.9 mm. These scopes can be easily passed transorally or transnasally, increasing the potential for sedationless endoscopy.(17) This modification will significantly reduce the direct and indirect costs of performing these procedures.

Small Bowel Endoscopy

Endoscopic visualization of the small bowel remains difficult. Three techniques currently exist: push enteroscopy, surgical endoscopy, and sonde enteroscopy.(17) In push enteroscopy, a long endoscope (typically a colonoscope or specifically designed enteroscope) is passed beyond the ligament of Treitz. An overtube is generally used to facilitate passage and prevent looping in the stomach. Push endoscopy generally does not allow visualization of the distal small bowel.(17) For surgical endoscopy, the entire small bowel is visualized. In this case, the surgeon manually advances the endoscope through the surgically exposed small intestine. In sonde enteroscopy, the tip of a small caliber enteroscope is allowed to passively move through the small intestine. The instrument is very flexible and very long (270-400 cm). This technique allows visualization of the distal small bowel, but has only diagnostic capabilities.(17)

Colonoscopy

Virtual colonoscopy, or more accurately computerized tomographic colography, involves the 3-D computerized reconstruction of images obtained by high-resolution helical computerized tomographic imaging.(17) The images are displayed on a video monitor, analogous to what is displayed during colonoscopy. The radiologist can electronically advance or withdraw the scope through the colon and search for pathology. Unfortunately, the sensitivity for polyp detection is not yet acceptable.(30)

Operative Approach
Laparoscopy

The laparoscopic alternative to conventional surgery has been an explosive area of growth in contemporary surgical practice. New techniques and procedures appear on a yearly, if not monthly basis. This revolution has been fueled by the beliefs of surgeons, referring physicians, and the general public that minimally invasive laparoscopic procedures entail less pain and lead to a faster recovery, compared to the conventional, "open" approach. There is already a large body of literature documenting the success of the laparoscopic approach, listing decreased requirements for post-operative pain medication, a decrease in the total number of hospital days, a faster return to work, and an overall improved quality of life following these procedures.(31, 32)

The laparoscopic approach is currently the preferred approach for cholecystectomy, inguinal and incisional/ventral herniorrhaphy, Nissen fundoplication, appendectomy, adrenalectomy and splenectomy. Surgeons are still awaiting significant technical advances which will allow them to easily perform small bowel, colonic and rectal procedures. While some of the current "cutting edge" practitioners are performing these small bowel and colonic procedures, this is not yet the standard of care. The use of the laparoscopic approach for the treatment of malignancy remains controversial and continues to be studied.

Further advances in the minimally invasive approach/robotics

The acceptance of laparoscopic techniques has changed the field of surgery in many regards. Further advances in technology and the "minimally invasive approach" will be necessary before surgeons will easily be able to perform the majority of gastrointestinal surgical procedures related to the small intestine and colon. Improvements in endoscopic vision systems and instrument functionality, as well as increases in the degrees of freedom of motion of the instruments will be necessary to perform increasingly complex procedures. Robotics will likely be the technologic future of laparoscopic surgery. Future technology will provide 3-D visualization, tactile sensation, and all degrees of freedom of motion for manipulation of surgical instruments, analogous to the human hand and wrist, reproducing the basic functional qualities that are characteristic of open surgery. Once this technology is achieved, this will allow many more gastrointestinal operative procedures to be performed in a "minimally invasive" fashion.

The "systems technology" associated with these advances will be key to facilitating the smooth flow of processes within the operating room. The integration of the different devices used for laparoscopic procedures into systems structures which are easy to control and maintain will be important for optimizing processes and resource allocations within the operating room. Operating rooms will need to integrate laparoscopic and robotic equipment with additional modalities for therapy, such as cryosurgery or radioablation probes and machines.

Concurrent with the advances in the minimally invasive approach to gastrointestinal surgery, other technologic advances may potentially allow for "virtual surgery." Telecommunications technologies applied to the surgical fields will leverage surgical expertise among centers, facilitate information transfer, and accelerate the diffusion and acceptance of surgical techniques among the leading medical centers. Telecommunications can be divided into 3 areas with respect to the treatment of surgical patients: teleconsulting, teleassistance, and telemanipulation.(33) Teleconsulting will likely enter the clinical realm in the near future, providing surgical consultation based on video transmitted from one center to another.

Teleassistance and telemanipulation require development before they become practical in the operating room. Teleassistance is defined as having a remote operator able to move and adjust the laparoscopic image to his or her needs. Telemanipulation will require significant advances in robotic technology that will allow manipulation of both the endoscopic camera and instruments by a remote operator.(33) Along with this explosion of technology, a careful analysis of the ethics associated with these techniques must occur. While technology may allow for significant advances in the surgical procedures that are available to patients, we must guard against compromising the physician-patient relationship.

Future Directions For Treatment Of Malignancies
Current state-of-the-art treatments
The current therapies for GI malignancies involve combined modalities.

Pancreatic Cancer
Pancreatic cancer represents only 2% of all malignancies, but is the fourth leading cause of cancer-related death in the United States.(34) While surgery remains the only curative treatment, the majority of patients with this disease are unresectable

at the time of presentation. There has been increasing success in pancreatic cancer treatment with combination chemotherapy, radiation therapy, and surgery. Recent studies have used a variety of chemotherapeutic agents, including 5-fluorouracil, gemcitabine, and cisplatin, in combination with radiation therapy.(35-37) Protocols have utilized both pre- and post-operative treatments. Although the studies to date are small, they do suggest that a combined modality approach is beneficial in the treatment of this disease process, increasing resectability rates as well as overall survival.(35-37)

Even with these new interventions and protocols, survival for this disease is dismal. A long term study of pancreatic cancer patients produced the following survival statistics: for patients undergoing resection versus no resection, median survival was 13.5 vs 3.1 months.(38) For resected patients, additional adjuvant therapy increased survival to 16.1 months versus 5.1 months for resected patients who received no additional treatment.(38) Survival in the setting of unresectable disease is particularly bleak; unresectable patients receiving chemoradiation treatment survived a median of 5.3 months versus 1.8 months for untreated and unresected patients.(38) Pathologic stage clearly has an impact on survival in pancreatic cancer: for patients who underwent surgical resection and had negative nodes, survival was 15% at 5 years versus 0% for resected patients with positive nodes.(38) Multimodality treatment clearly improves survival for patients with pancreatic cancer; however, we have a long way to go to reach satisfactory treatment results for this type of GI cancer.

Gastric Cancer

Treatment for gastric cancer remains disappointing. Surgical resection offers the only opportunity for cure, but this is rarely successful as the majority of these patients present late in the disease course. Combined modality treatments with chemotherapy, radiation therapy, and surgery also produce relatively poor results, making this one of the more difficult GI cancers to treat. While there has been some recent success with combined modality therapy for pancreatic and colorectal cancers, similar successes for gastric malignancies have not been observed.

Colorectal Cancer

Aside from treatment of the earliest stages of colorectal cancer, therapy for this type of malignancy includes chemotherapy, radiation therapy, and surgery, not necessarily in that order. For example, a study from the Swedish Rectal Cancer Trial demonstrated improved local control and survival in rectal cancer patients treated with a short course of high-dose preoperative radiotherapy as compared with patients treated with surgery alone (58% versus 48% overall 5 year survival, p=0.004).(39)

For patients with isolated hepatic metastases from colorectal cancer, surgical resection, offers the best option for cure. Intra-operative ultrasound (IOUS) is now an important adjunct in the surgical treatment of hepatic colorectal metastases. The use of IOUS to image the liver in patients who were being explored for a planned hepatic resection modified the operative management of 44% of the patients studied.(40)

Additional treatment modalities, including cryotherapy and radiofrequency ablation, are increasingly utilized to manage patients with isolated hepatic colorectal metastases. Several studies have suggested that cryoablation and/or radiofrequency ablation may provide equivalent results to hepatic resection in these patients. Cryotherapy destroys cells directly as a result of physiochemical effects and indirectly by obliteration of tumor vessels, causing hypoxia and necrosis. The technique can be used for multiple liver lesions, for bilobar disease, as an aid to segmental resection, and in those patients with poor hepatic reserve or comorbid conditions that preclude major hepatic resection. The treatment of hepatic colorectal metastases with cryotherapy has resulted in similar cure rates to that seen with resective therapy.(41) This new technology has allowed some patients who would have previously been considered unresectable to be "resected" with cryosurgery for cure. Laparoscopic ultrasonography and laparoscopic cryotherapy have been combined successfully. This combination of technologies may result in less post-operative morbidity in patients being treated for "unresectable" hepatic metastases.(42)

Radiofrequency ablation (RFA) is a similar technique to cryoablation, but uses heat rather than cold, to obliterate tumors. Its efficacy and uses are similar to cryotherapy and the technique can also be used laparoscopically. Cryotherapy and radiofrequency ablative techniques have been used in combination, with the use of RFA reducing the morbidity of multiple freezes.(43) RFA is limited by tumor size (<3 cm).

For patients with isolated colorectal hepatic metastases, surgical resection offers the best chance for cure. Recent data suggests that survival in resected patients may be improved with the addition of chemotherapy. The combination of hepatic resection with hepatic arterial infusion pump placement for chemotherapy administration offers improved survival and increase quality of life for patients with hepatic colorectal metastases; in one study, survival free of hepatic recurrence at two years was improved from 60% to 90% by combining resection with intra-arterial hepatic chemotherapy.(44) Although the follow up in this study was short, it does suggest an important effect of combined therapy, that regional chemotherapy is more effective than systemic chemotherapy for liver-only metastases due to colorectal cancer.

Hepatocellular Carcinoma (HCC)

The treatment of hepatocellular carcinoma is often more difficult than that of other types of hepatic neoplasms and overall survival for this tumor remains poor. Hepatocellular carcinoma (HCC) commonly occurs in a background of cirrhosis, limiting hepatic reserve and ability to tolerate aggressive therapies poor. Resection is reserved for patients with solitary HCC who have adequate hepatic reserve, and is the only treatment modality that offers a reasonable hope of disease-free survival.

In light of the above issues, HCC is commonly treated with other modalities. Ethanol injection may be used; it has a good efficacy at treating the local tumor and is often amenable to percutaneous administration under ultrasound guidance. This technique is highly effective for solitary tumors less than 3 cm; 90% of these lesions undergo complete necrosis.(45) The success rate in larger tumors is significantly less, and even for smaller tumors in which complete necrosis occurs, HCC recurrence is frequent.(45) The recurrence rate and patterns are similar to those seen following resection, and this treatment produces similar survival rates to that of resective therapy.(45)

HCC has also been treated with chemoembolization. This therapy combines obstruction of arterial flow to the area of the tumor with the injection of chemotherapeutic agents suspended in lipiodol (a contrast agent that is selectively retained in the tumor). Ischemic necrosis generally affects more than 80% of the HCC in the majority of patients treated with this technique.(45) Unfortunately, despite initial studies which showed tumor necrosis, no survival benefit has been demonstrated in prospective studies.(45) Treatment with radiotherapy, chemotherapy, and hormonal manipulations has also been disappointing.(45) Despite advances in multimodality treatment for many types of GI tumors, treatment for HCC remains difficult with low success rates.

Until the genetics and cellular mechanisms of cancer are elucidated to the level where they can be manipulated and controlled, cancer treatment will likely encompass continued combined modality therapies, including the surgeon, radiation therapist, medical oncologist, and interventional radiologist.

Specific treatments aimed at the molecular basis of carcinogenesis

Understanding of the genetic and cellular mechanisms underlying malignancy, are progressing at an astounding rate. Although specific, directed treatments have not yet come forward, there are several promising areas. A new pharmacologic agent, Gleevac (imatinib mesylate), which is a protein-kinase inhibitor, has demonstrated remarkable effectiveness at initiating GI stromal tumor regression. In vitro studies using this agent have demonstrated that it is not entirely selective; it also inhibits the tyrosine receptor kinases for platelet-derived growth factor and stem cell factor and its receptor, c-kit, inhibiting the cellular events initiated by these factors.(46) This relatively targeted therapy has proven very effective in early trials against gastrointestinal stromal tumors, resulting in significant tumor regression.(46)

Anti-angiogenesis agents may also have significant impact on the treatment of epithelial malignancies. Although anti-angiogenesis cancer therapies initially appeared promising, further investigations have shown that this therapy may be highly effective as long as it is specifically tailored to the type of malignancy being treated. A recent study by Kuo and coworkers investigated the relative potency of several anti-angiogenesis gene products administered via recombinant adenoviruses against various types of tumors.(47) The relative effectiveness of angiostatin, endostatin, neuropilin and the ligand-binding ectodomains of the vascular endothelial growth factor receptors, delivered via recombinant adenoviruses in several different murine tumor models was studied.(47) These investigations documented that the ectodomains of the vascular endothelial growth factor receptors were highly effective at inhibiting tumor growth (80% inhibition) in murine models of lung carcinoma, fibrosarcoma, and pancreatic carcinoma.(47) In contrast, viral delivery of angiostatin, endostatin, and neuropilin were significantly less effective in these tumor models.(47)

Another promising concept is that of "suicide gene therapy". While yet to be clinically tested, some promising laboratory results have been obtained. In these investigations, "suicide genes" are transferred into tumor cells. The most common suicide gene codes for the herpes simplex type I thymidine kinase, which converts nontoxic nucleoside analogs, such as ganciclovir, into toxic triphosphated compounds. In animal studies, rats with tumors which underwent retroviral-mediated transfer of these "suicide genes" were treated with ganciclovir with significant reduction in tumor burden.(48)

While currently in its infancy, the use of microarray technologies to monitor gene expression in model organisms, cell lines, and human tissues has become an important part of biological research over the last several years.(49-51) This technology will likely become important in clinical medicine in the future, particularly for the diagnosis and treatment of malignancies. Oligonucleotide-directed microarrays are highly sensitive, quantitative, and comparisons are possible across many tissues and samples. This technology is particularly useful for the molecular profiling of various cancers, providing information regarding the molecular characteristics of the cancer under study.(51-53) Oligonucleotide-directed microarrays can distinguish between closely related cancer subtypes and gene profiling can help to identify groups of genes involved in specific functional aspects of tumor biology.(53-55)

Trends in Medical Education in GI Surgery
Laparoscopic training

For many advanced laparoscopic procedures, including Nissen fundoplication, inguinal and ventral/incisional herniorrhaphy, splenectomy, and adrenalectomy, a significant learning curve has been documented.(56-58) Generally, these procedures require more training and practice than the simpler procedures, such as laparoscopic cholecystectomy. The problems with adequacy of training for laparoscopic procedures are underscored by documented increases in morbidity and mortality associated with these procedures.(59) The State of New York has recently implemented standards for the credentialing and performance of laparoscopic cholecystectomy.(59) Advanced forms of training are available and include laparoscopic virtual reality simulators; unfortunately, these simulators are not yet lifelike and their cost is significant.(60) Telemedicine mentoring and assistance is also a possible avenue for additional training, particularly for the surgeon who is already in practice. Medicolegal issues and scheduling constraints have not yet allowed this practice to be easily implemented.(61) Multi-media interactive computer-based training is a tool that is widely utilized by the military, as well as the high tech industries in the business world. This form of training has been shown to decrease learning curves by 60% and to increase retention by 50% when compared to traditional didactic methods.(59,62) This technique has been shown to facilitate the acquisition of laparoscopic skills, particularly when combined with more traditional didactic and hands-on laboratory training experiences.(59)

In the very near future, there will be a set "curriculum" for the acquisition of laparoscopic skills. Surgical residents will be required to practice in a surgical skills laboratory and to document that they have achieved the necessary technical skills prior to coming to the operating room. Although curriculums will be focused on the acquisition of laparoscopic skills, additional laboratory-based training in other basic surgical skills, such as suturing, knot typing, and stapling will be developed in this context as well. While the operating room is often an excellent "classroom", the acquisition of certain key surgical skills prior to entering the operating room will lessen the stress involved in the learning process. Decreases in stress levels have been shown to enhance learning. In addition, skills acquisition may also decrease operating room times for various procedures, increasing cost effectiveness and overall quality of patient care. There will be increased space needs to supply a "Surgical Skills Training Laboratory," appropriately equipped with the necessary tools for resident training. In addition, residents and faculty alike will need adequate time for training and practicing purposes. In the future, technology will likely become an even larger part of surgical practice, including the use of robotics and telemedicine. It is critical that training programs keep pace with these technological advances.

Emphasis on Having a Curriculum with Measured Competencies and Standards of Performance in All Resident Training Programs

The American Council for Graduate Medical Education has mandated that all residency programs begin to integrate learning objectives and evaluation tools into their training programs. The Council has mandated that by July, 2002 all residency programs will document resident competence in six different core areas.(Table 5) These competencies reflect the organization's interpretation of what society expects from a competent physician.

Table 5. General Competencies as outlined by the ACGME

Patient Care, which is compassionate, appropriate, and effective for the treatment of health problems and the promotion of health

Medical Knowledge about established and evolving biomedical, clinical and cognate sciences and the application of this knowledge to patient care

Practice-based learning and improvement that involves investigation and evaluation of their own patient care, appraisal, and assimilation of scientific evidence and improvements in patient care

Interpersonal and communication skills that result in effective information exchange and learning with patients, their families, and other health professionals

Professionalism as manifested through a commitment to carrying out professional responsibilities, adherence to ethical principles, and sensitivity to a diverse patient population

Systems-based practice as manifested by actions that demonstrate an awareness of and response to the larger context and system of health careand effectively call on system resources to provide optimal care.

While the current emphasis on curriculum and competencies is at the medical student and resident level, it is likely that this process will eventually include all surgeons. Patients have become active participants in their own health care and demand accurate information regarding options for treatment and outcomes. Patient satisfaction has become an important component of the provision of medical care. For most patients, the patriarchal physician is no longer appreciated. Physicians need to partner with their patients in order to provide the best care.

Practice Trends
Documentation of Competence

The American Board of Surgery (ABS) has strongly endorsed the American Board of Medical Specialties Competence Initiative by committing itself to the concept of maintaining the certification of its members (63), seeking to link ABS certification with competence in practice, and ensuring that certified individuals possess at all times, the same qualifications that were present on the day that the certificate was issued. It has becoming increasingly important for physicians and surgeons to demonstrate continued evidence of life-long learning practices, a continuous highly professional behavior, periodic self-assessment, continuous cognitive expertise, and continuous self-evaluation of performance in practice. It is likely that some evaluation of outcomes will be undertaken as part of this process. It is also highly likely that this process will become more rigorous over time, with physicians and surgeons being required to document competence and life-long learning throughout their careers.

The Physician-Patient Relationship

The changes in the structure and financing of the health care system have significantly stressed the surgeon-patient relationship, weakening the essential trust that is necessary to this liaison. As technology increases, it is the surgeon's goal and obligation to continue to strengthen the physician-patient relationship, by maintaining good communication and advocating for his or her patients. Because many insurers utilize capitation or other cost control strategies to shift the financial risk of health service utilization to the providers as a means of insuring cost-effective care, this linkage between financing and provision of services can potentially lead to withholding of appropriate services, creating a conflict between a physician's financial interest and the patient's clinical interest. There is an increasing emphasis on continued competence for practicing physicians and surgeons. There will likely be an increased emphasis placed on results, outcomes, and overall patient satisfaction in order to maintain a healthy referral base. Hopefully, a logical and rational approach to this problem will be undertaken, lest this scrutiny drive surgeons away from complex, seriously ill patients due to concerns regarding the impact of poor outcomes on their practice. For example, recent studies have suggested improved outcomes for many complex procedures in hospitals which perform higher volumes. For Whipple procedures, a 3 to 4-fold increase for in-hospital mortality rates has been documented for hospitals which perform a low- to very low-volume of this procedure.(64) This type of analysis of procedurally related outcomes is increasing and will likely determine where patients seek treatment in the future.

REFERENCES

1.   Wilmoth JR, Timiras PS. Demography of aging; comparative, differential, and successful aging; geriatric assessment. In: Principles and Practice of Geriatric Surgery. Rosenthal RA, Zenilman ME, and Katlic MR, eds. Springer-Verlag, NY, 2001 pgs. 24-37.

2.   Palmer RM. Acute care. In: Principles of Geriatric Medicine and Gerontology. Hazard WR, Blass JP, Ettinger WH, Halter JB, Ouslander JG, eds. McGraw-Hill, New York, NY, 1999 pgs. 483-492.

3. Walter LC, Brand RJ, Counsell SR, Palmer RM, Landefeld CS, Fortinsky RH, Covinsky KE. Development and validation of a prognostic index for 1-year mortality in older adults after hospitalization. JAMA 2001 285:2987-2994.

4. Yancik R, Ries LA. Cancer in older persons: Magnitude of the problem-how do we apply what we know? Cancer. 1994 74:1995-2003.

5. Blair SL, Schwarz RE. Advanced age does not contribute to increased risks or poor outcome after major abdominal operations. Am Surg 2001 67;1123-1127.

6. DiCarlo V, Balzano G, Zerni A, Villa E. Pancreatic cancer resection in elderly patients. Br J Surg 1998 85:607-610.

7. Begg CB, Cramer LD, Hoskins WJ, Brennan MF. Impact of hospital volume on operative mortality for major cancer surgery (see comments). JAMA 1998 280:1747-1751.

8. Brink JA, McFarland EG, Heiken JP. Helical/spiral computer body tomography. Clin Radiol 1997 52:489-503.

9. Ferrucci JT. Advances in abdominal MR imaging. Radiographics 1998 18:1569-1586.

10. Ademek HE, Breer H, Karschkes T, Albert J, Reimann JF. Magnetic resonance imaging in gastroenterology: time to say good bye to all that endoscopy? Endoscopy 2000 32:406-410.

11. Vitellas KM, Keogan MT, Spritzer CE, Nelson RC. MR cholangiopancreatography of bile and pancreatic duct abnormalities with emphasis on single-shot fast spin-echo technique. Radiographics 2000 20:939-957.

12. Hochwald SH, Rofsky NM, Dobryansky M, Shamamian P, Marcus SG. Magnetic resonance imaging with magnetic resonance cholangiopancreatography accurately predicts the resectability of pancreatic carcinoma. J Gastrointest Surg 1999 3:506-511.

13. Rajput A, Stellato TA, Faulhader PF, Vesselle HJ, Miraldi F. The role of fluorodeoxyglucose emission tomography in the evaluation of pancreatic disease. Surgery 1998 124:793-798.

14. Delbeke D, Martin WH, Sandler MP, Chapman WC, Wright K, Pinson CW. Evaluation of benign vs malignant hepatic lesions with positron emission tomography. Arch Surg 1998 133:510-516.

15. Strasberg SM, Dehdashti F, Siegel BA, Drebin JA, Linenan D. Survival of patients evaluated by FDG-PET before hepatic resection for metastatic colorectal carcinoma: A prospective database study. Ann Surg 2001 233:293-299.

16. Huebner RH, Park KC, Shepard JS, Schwimmer J, Czernin J, Phelps ME, Gambhirr SS. A meta-analysis of the literature for whole body FDG-PET detection of recurrent colorectal cancer. J Nucl Med 2000 41:1177-1189.

17. Mallery S, Van Dam J. Endoscopic practice at the start of the new millennium. Gastro 2000 118:S129-S147.

18. Yasuda K, Mukai H, Nakajima M. Endoscopic ultrasonography diagnosis of pancreatic cancer. Gastrointest Endosc Clin North Am 1995 5:699-712.

19. Chak A, Canto MI Rosch T, Dittler HJ, Hawes RH, Tio TL, Lightdale CJ, Boyce HW, Scheiman J, Carpenter SL, Van Dam J, Kochman ML, Sivak MV Jr. Endoscopic differentiation of benign and malignant stromal cell tumors. Gastrointest Endosc 1997 45:468-473.

20. Mallery S, DeCamp M, Bueno R, Mentzer SJ, Sugarbaker DJ, Swanson SJ, Van Dam J. Pretreatment staging by endoscopic ultrasonography does not predict complete response to neoadjuvant chemoradiation in patients with esophageal carcinoma. Cancer 1999 86:764-769.

21. Wiersema MJ, Wiersema LM. Endosonographically-guided celiac plexus neurolysis. Gastrointest Endosc 1996 44:656-662.

22. Brugge WR. Endoscopic ultrasonography: The current status. Gastro 1998 115:1577-1583.

23. Fosmark CE. Differential diagnosis of pancreatic tumors. Gastrointest Endosc Clin North Am 1995 5;713-721.

24. Rosch T. Staging of pancreatic cancer: analysis of literature results. Gastrointest Endosc Clin North Am 1995 5:735-739.

25. Brugge WR, Lee MJ, Kelsey PB, Schapiro RH, Warshaw AL. The use of EUS to diagnose malignant portal venous system invasion by pancreatic cancer. Gastrointest Endosc 1996 43:561-567.

26. Legmann P, Vignaux O, Dousset B, Baraza AJ, Palazzo L, Dumontier I, Coste J, Louvel A, Roseau G, Couturier D, Bonnin A. Pancreatic tumors: comparison of dual-phase helical CT and endoscopic sonography. Am J Roentgenol 1998 170:1315-1322.

27. Van Dam J. Endosonography of the esophagus. Gastrointest Endosc Clin North Am 1994;803-826.

28. Lightdale CJ. Detection of anastomotic recurrence of endoscopic ultrasonography. Gastrointest Clin North Am 1995 5:595-600.

29. Dershaw D, Enker W, Cohen AM, Sigurdson E. Transrectal ultrasonography of rectal carcinoma. Cancer 1990 66:2336-2340.

30. Rex DK, Vining D, Kopecky KK. An initial experience with screening for colorectal polyps using spiral CT with and without CT colography. Gastrointest Endo 1999 49:566-565.

31. Filipi CJ, Gaston-Johansson F, McBride PJ, Murayama Y, Gerhardt J, Cornet DA, Lund RJ, Hirai D, Graham R, Patil K, Fitzgibbons R Jr, Gaines RD. An assessment of pain and return to normal activity: Laparoscopic herniorrhaphy vs open tension-free Lichtenstein repair. Surg Endo 1996 10:983-986.

32. Velanovich V. Laparoscopic vs open surgery: A preliminary comparison of quality-of-life outcomes. Surg Endo 2000 14:16-21.

33. Schurr MO, Arezzo A, Buess GF. Robotics and systems technology for advanced endoscopic procedures: experiences in general surgery. Eur J Cardio-Thor Surg 1999 16(Suppl 2):S97-S105.

34. Landis SH, Murray T, Bolden S, Wingo PA. Cancer Statistics 1999 CA Cancer J Clin 1999 44:8-34.

35. Mehta VK, Fisher G, Ford JA, Poen JC, Vierra MA, Oberhelman H, Niederhuber J, Bastidas JA. Preoperative chemoradiation for marginally resectable adenocarcinoma of the pancreas. J Gastrointest Surg 2001 5:27-35.

36. Wanebo HJ, Glicksman AS, Vezeridis MP, Clark J, Tibbetts L, Koness J, Levy A. Preoperative chemotherapy, radiotherapy, and surgical resection of locally advanced pancreatic cancer. Arch Surg 2000 135:81-87.

37. White RR, Hurwitz HI, Mors MA, Lee C, Anscher MS, Paulson EK, Gottfried MR, Baillie J, Branch MS, Jowell PS, McGrath KM, Clary BM, Pappas TN, Tyler DS. Neoadjuvant chemoradiation for localized adenocarcinoma of the pancreas. Ann Surg Oncol 2001 8:758-765.

38. Carr JA, Ajlouni M, Wollner I, Wong D, Velanovich V. Adenocarcinoma of the head of the pancreas: Effects of surgical and nonsurgical therapy on survival-A ten year experience. Am Surg 1999 65:1143-1149.

39. Swedish Rectal Cancer Trial. Improved survival with preoperative radiotherapy in resectable rectal cancer. NEJM 1997 336:980-987.

40. Cervone A, Sardi A, Conaway GL. Intraoperative ultrasound (IOUS) is essential in the management of metastatic colorectal liver lesions. Am Surg 2000 66:611-615.

41. Wallace JR, Christians KK, Pitt HA, Quebbeman EJ. Cryotherapy extends the indications for treatment of colorectal liver metastases. Surgery 1999 126:766-774.

42. Iannitti DA, Heniford BT, Hale J, Grundfest-Broniatowski S, Ganger M. Laparoscopic cryoablation of hepatic metastases. Arch Surg 1998 133:1011-1015.

43. Bilchik AJ, Wood TF, Allegra D, Tsiolias GJ, Chung M, Rose M, Ramming KP, Morton DL. Cryosurgical ablation and radiofrequency ablation for unresectable hepatic malignant neoplasms. Arch Surg 2000 135:657-664.

44. Kemeny N, Huang Y, Cohen AM, Shi W, Conti JA, Brennan MF, Bertina JR, Turnbull ADM, Sullivan D, Stockman J, Blumgart LH, Fong Y. Hepatic arterial infusion of chemotherapy after resection of hepatic metastases from colorectal cancer. NEJM 1999 341:2039-2048.

45. Bruix J. Treatment of hepatocellular carcinoma. Hepatol 1997 25:259-262.

46. Berman J, O'Leary TJ. Gastrointestinal stromal tumor workshop. Hum Path 2001 6:578-582.

47. Kuo CJ, Farnebo F, Yu E, Christofferson R, Swearingen RA, Carter R, von Recum HA, Yuan J, Kamihara J, Flynn E, D'Amato R, Folkman J, Mulligan RC. Comparative evaluation of the antitumor activity of antiangiogenic proteins delivered by gene transfer. Proc Nat Acad of Sci USA 2001 98:4605-4610.

48. Nagy H, Panis Y, Fabre M, Perrin H, Klatzmann D, Houssin D. Are hepatomas a good target for suicide gene therapy? An experimental study in rats using retroviral-mediated transfer of thymidine kinase gene. Surgery 1998 123:19-24.

49. Cho RJ, Fromont-Racine M, Wodicka L, Feierbach B, Stearns T, Legrain P, Lockhart DJ, Eavis RW. Parallel analysis of genetic selections using whole genome oligonucleotide arrays. Proc Nat Acad Sci USA 1998 95:3752-3757.

50. deVeer MJ, Holko M, Frevel M, Walker E, Der S, Paranjape JM, Silverman RH, Williams BR. Functional classification of interferon-stimulated genes identified using microarrays. J Leuk Biol 2001 69:912-920.

51. Notterman DA, Alon U, Sierk AJ, Levine AJ. Transcriptional gene expression profiles of colorectal adenoma, adenocarcinoma, and normal tissue examined by oligonucleotide arrays. Cancer Res 2001 61:3124-3130.

52. DeRisi J, Penland L, Brown PO, Bittner ML, Meltzer PS, Ray M, Chen Y, SuYA, Trent JM. Use of a cDNA microarray to analyse gene expression patterns in human cancer. Nat Genet 1996 14:457-460.

53. Welsh JB, Zarrinkar PP, Sapinsos LM, Kern SG, Behling CA, Monk BJ, Lockhart DJ, Burger RA, Hampton GM. Analysis of gene expression profiles in normal and neoplastic ovarian tissue samples identifies candidate molecular markers of epithelial ovarian cancer. Proc Natl Acad Sci USA 2001 98:1176-1181.

54. Califano A, Stolovitzky G, Tu Y. Analysis of gene expression microarrays for phenotype classification. Pro Int Conf Intell Syst Mol Biol 2000 8:75-85.

55. Gutgemann A, Golob M, Muller S, Buettner R, Bosserhoff AK. Isolation of invasion-associated cDNAs in melanoma. Arch Dermatol Res 2001 293:282-290.

56. Watson DI, Baigrie RJ, Jamieson GG. A learning curve for laparoscopic fundoplication: definable, avoidable, or a waste of time? Ann Surg 1996 224:198-203.

57. Wright D, O'Dwyer PJ. The learning curve for laparoscopic hernia repair. Semin Laparosc Surg 1998 5:227-232.

58. Way LW. General surgery in evolution: technology and competence. Am J Surg 1996 171:2-8.

59. Ramshaw BJ, Young D, Garcha I, Shuler F, Wilson R, White JG, Duncan T, Mason E. The role of multimedia interactive programs in training for laparoscopic procedures. Surg Endo 2001 15:21-27.

60. Satava RM, Krusch DA. Computers in surgery: telesurgery, virtual reality, and the new world order of medicine. Contemp Surg 1995 47:204-208.

61. Rosser JC, Wood M, Payne JH, Fullum TM, Lisehora GB, Rosser LE, Barcia PJ, Savalgi RS. Telementoring: a practical option in surgical training. Surg Endo 1997 11:852-855.

62. Rosser J. CD-ROM multimedia: the next step before virtual reality. Surg Endo 1996 10:1033-1035.

63. Ritchie WP Jr. The measurement of competence: current plans and future initiatives of the American Board of Surgery. Bull Am Coll Surgeons 2001 86:5-10.

64. Birkmeyer JD, Finlayson SRG, Tosteson ANA, Sharp SM, Warshaw AL, Fisher ES. Effect of hospital volume on in-hospital mortality with pancreaticoduodenectomy. Surgery 1999 125:250-256.

CHAPTER 11

ORTHOPEDIC SURGERY

ANDREW A. FREIBERG, M.D.

The future of orthopedic surgery is extraordinarily bright, with remarkable changes in store that will advance our abilities to provide restoration of function and lifetime disease management. Only fifty years ago, orthopedic surgeons used mould arthroplasty as a technique to replace part of an arthritic hip joint. Sir John Charnley developed the low friction arthroplasty in the early 1960s and this concept revolutionized treatment of hip arthritis. Despite the acclaim of this new technique in England, most of the subsequent improvements in materials and technique have taken place in the United States. These advances have made the procedures among the most successful, durable and cost-effective in the past century.

In the early 1900s, orthopedic surgeons focused on musculoskeletal sepsis, the sequelae of polio, congenital diseases such as clubfoot, scoliosis, rickets, and to lesser degrees, arthritis. Modern practices focus on surgical treatments for arthritis, trauma surgery, ligament and cartilage surgery of virtually all joints, minimally invasive procedures, outpatient surgery, and treatment of spinal disorders including herniated disks and degenerative arthritis. Musculoskeletal sepsis is now more often related to implants than spontaneous joint infections.

Advances in orthopedic surgery have centered on restoration of function through either repair or reconstruction. Surgical reconstruction of diseased joints has evolved from simple debridements in the early part of the 1900s into sophisticated joint replacements. Joint replacement (arthroplasty) has become one of the most successful and cost effective surgical procedures performed. Hip arthroplasty is more cost-effective than coronary artery bypass grafts, liver or kidney transplantation, and vascular bypass procedures.

Total Hip Arthroplasty

When total hip arthroplasty was invented, there were severe material limitations that led to early implant failure. The acetabular components were initially made from Teflon as investigators assumed low friction and low wear were crucial. The femoral components were made from lower quality stainless steel and the incidence of stem fracture was approximately one percent. There have been advances in bone cementing techniques, implant design, and development of porous ingrowth surfaces so that bone can bond directly to prosthesis. Future implants will show substantial advances in design and new materials that may be far different from the currently employed metals, ceramics and plastics. The problems of predictable skeletal fixation have been addressed in the past 10 years, but yet to be solved is the materials problem: wear of the articulation between the artificial femoral head and the plastic liner of the acetabulum.

The recent introduction of highly crosslinked ultra-high molecular weight polyethylene (XLPE) is one of the most significant advances in total hip arthroplasty to date. These so-called alternate bearing surfaces are attempts to decrease wear at the articulation and extend the longevity of the replacement. The goal is to have a lifetime arthroplasty of such quality that the indications can be extended to younger patients. There are a number of currently available alternate bearing surfaces including XLPE, ceramics, specially treated metals (e.g. nitrogen ion hardened), and metal-on-metal articulations.

Assessing methods for these new articulations is a complex process involving materials and biocompatibility testing, wear simulation and tribologic testing. Current methods for wear simulation are a dramatic advance over prior methods and as our knowledge of joint kinetics and kinematics improves, the testing will improve as well. Testing methods for most polyethylenes included simple pin on disc wear testing and simple arc range of motions under a fixed load. The testing was often performed using water as a lubricant. These methods are no longer accepted as valid due to lack of physiologic simulation and inability to predict clinical performance and implant retrieval findings. A hip simulator has recently been developed to test new materials for hip replacement.(Figure 1) This device evaluates the implants using physiologic loads relevant to walking and stair climbing and includes the critical elements of crossing pathways. A new highly cross-linked ultrahigh molecular weight polyethylene developed recently and tested with this device shows virtually no wear when tested up to 20 million cycles, with low wear independent of femoral head size. Because of this finding, the FDA has recently approved the clinical use of large femoral heads, up to 40 mm. This increase in articulation size allows for improved hip joint range of motion accompanied by a logarithmic improvement in joint stability.

The amount of linear and volumetric wear from migration of the femoral head is extremely important. This wear produces billions of submicron particles that can lead to bone resorption (osteolysis) and also to implant loosening. The wear of XLPE is so low that routine methods used for radiographic measurement do not work. With standard non-crosslinked polyethylenes, the annual wear rate of most total hip arthroplastics is approximately 0.1 – 0.2 mm per year but plain radiographs can only detect alteration to an accuracy of 0.5 mm. Because XLPEs wear so little, new methods are being utilized that can reproducibly measure changes as small as 0.1 mm. This method employs 2 simultaneously performed orthogonal radiographs and 0.1 mm tantalum beads implanted in the acetabular liner.(Figure 2) Only this type of detailed study will define the future best articulation.

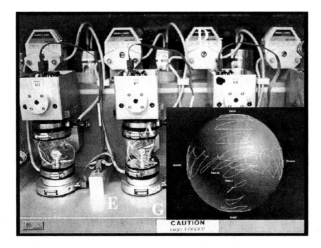

Figure 11-1

Hip Simulator. This device precisely models normal human gait and stairclimbing to evaluate wear and implant function in new devices before they are ever implanted in humans. The overlay in the right corner shows a polar diagram of the crossing pathways during normal gait.

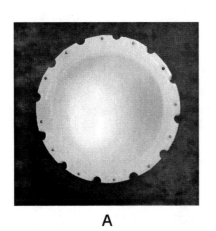

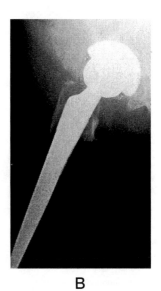

A

B

Figure 11-2

(A) Acetabular polyethylene and (B) radiograph demonstrates the tantalum beads used to accurately measure polyethylene wear and implant movement.

Much attention has been given to other alternate bearing surfaces, and especially ceramic on ceramic articulations. These have extremely low wear, but there are technical issues with implantation (chipping and fracture of the liner at insertion), a higher incidence of dislocation due to mechanical impingement, and catastrophic spontaneous fracture of the femoral head. This latter complication never occurs with modern metal femoral heads so any possible benefits from improved ceramic wettability and smoothness have not proved clinically relevant in over 10 years of use. Metal on metal articulations have also been tried with variable success. When manufactured with extreme care to provide proper femoral head clearance, these implants can have wear rates in the microns over many years. However, there are problems with these articulations including recent reports of delayed metal hypersensitivity and public health concerns about long term exposure to cobalt and chromium metal ions produced from wear. Although the wear rates are only microns, the number of metal ions released is in the billions and these concentrate in lymph nodes, local tissues and spleen. Concerns about carcinogenesis will likely limit the wider application of the devices in the future.

There have also been remarkable advances in surgical techniques for implantation of new joints. Orthopedic surgeons now routinely implant new hip joints through smaller incisions (10-15 cm) and very recent developments allow total hip arthroplasty utilizing two separate 2-3 cm incisions. The surgical dissection is so limited that some of these patients are allowed to go home within one day. For hip arthroplasty, these techniques are in their infancy and it will require prospective clinical trials to ensure safety and equivalent efficacy (similar rates of complication, loosening, and long term success). The technique for minimally invasive arthroplasty is highly dependent on successful intra-operative imaging. This fundamental change in technique will have profound effects on operating room designs for the future.

Knee Arthroplasty

There have been similar technique changes in knee arthroplasty. Recent clinical studies have demonstrated the long-term clinical success of partial knee replacement. Osteoarthritis can affect one or all three compartments of the knee (medial, lateral or patello-femoral). When arthritis is limited to one compartment, partial knee replacement is an option. Because only one condyle is resurfaced, the common term for this procedure is unicondylar arthroplasty. In the past year, a new surgical technique has been developed that allows unicondylar replacement through an 8 centimeter incision with a small arthrotomy.(Figure 3) This minimally invasive technique is radically different from the larger exposure necessary for total knee arthroplasty.(Figure 4) Patients with a unicondylar arthroplasty usually are discharged to home within 1 – 2 days and attain normal range of motion within 2 weeks. Most patients are able to return to office or professional work within two weeks. Standard knee replacement patients typically require an additional month of physical therapy, have

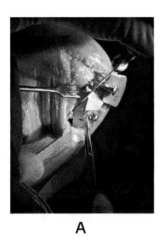

A

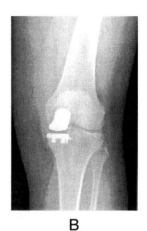

B

Figure 11-3

(A) Intra-operative view of minimally invasive unicondylar knee arthroplasty. (B) radiograph of a unicondylar arthroplasty

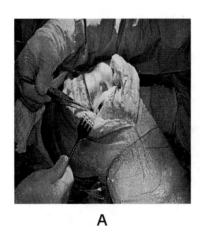

A

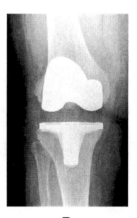

B

Figure 11-4

(A) Intra-operative view of standard total knee arthroplasty. (B) radiograph of a total knee replacement

more difficulty attaining normal range of motion and experience greater swelling and pain. Patient satisfaction with a less painful procedure, shorter hospitalization and earlier return to normal function has been the driving force in the development of these techniques.

There are ongoing efforts to develop total knee implants that can accommodate normal full range of motion without instability, mechanical impingement, or undue wear. The recent release of high flexion knee implants may lead to improved range of motion and function. These implants are designed to maintain femoral contact with the polyethylene insert so as to prevent increased localized posterior wear and also maintain cam/post interactions that improve stability when flexion is past 120 degrees.(Figure 5)

Similar to the improvements made in hip wear simulation, the recent introduction of robotic testing has changed our approach to total knee arthroplasty evaluation. Accurate robotic kinematic studies allow precise testing to optimize implant design and ultimately improve clinical range of motion.(Figure 6) Highly cross-linked ultra-high molecular weight polyethylenes will be introduced into the knee market in the near future. Early laboratory studies have demonstrated potential benefits using this new material in knee arthroplasty.

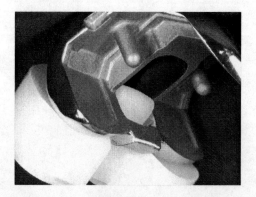

Figure 11-5
Photograph of a new high flexion total knee device

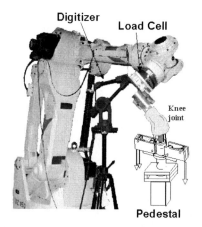
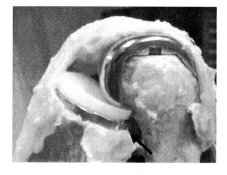

Digitizer
Load Cell
Knee joint
Pedestal

Lateral side at 150 deg.

Figure 11-6
Testing of a new robotic device for knee arthroplasty

Role of Robots

Intra-operative utilization of robots may be an important area for future development. The utility of robots is directly related to surgical navigation technology. A robot can only be as precise as its known position in space relative to the patient's unique anatomy. Early attempts at intra-operative robotics were related to precise machining of the femoral canal as preparation for cementless devices. The robots were able to accurately machine the canal, however there were periodic catastrophic fractures as the robot did not have sufficiently accurate navigation or "position sense", and was not able to respond independently to cues that would alert a surgeon to slow down or slightly adjust the angle of reaming. Robots will likely develop into highly capable assistants and work in the hands of skilled surgeons to perform some tasks more accurately, and allow for truly minimally invasive techniques.

Orthopedic surgeons are less than a decade away from robotically assisted arthroplastyutilizing one or two 1 cm incisions. One of the great challenges for the future will be surgical education training in the use of haptic robots. Surgical navigation techniques have evolved to a current level of usefulness for spinal surgery (placement of pedicle screws) and hip arthroplasty (acetabular component orientation). These types of navigation still require high quality CT scans of the target area. Novel methods for precise anatomic localization will need to be developed. The future will include new techniques such as functional micro-positioning systems. These will need to be installed in the operating rooms of the future and will likely require large capital expenditures.

Tissue Transplantation

Tissue transplantation is an integral aspect of modern orthopedic surgery. There are a number of commonly transplanted tissues used to reconstruct torn anterior cruciate ligaments, restore cancellous bone loss from osteolysis, replace segments of bone removed as part of tumor resections, and to treat bone loss from trauma, infection and osteonecrosis. This section will focus on allograft transplantation and future developments. In the United States, the most commonly transplanted tissues are for orthopedic reconstruction, with an incidence at least an order of magnitude greater than solid organ transplants.

Orthopedic surgeons are also encountering more severe bone loss associated with repeated joint arthroplasties as earlier implant designs and polyethylene continue to fail. These patients can require massive bulk allografts for reconstruction to restore ambulation and prevent amputation.(Figure 7) The biology of host-allograft interactions is extremely complex and improved understanding is vital since the allograft tissue must heal to the host. Current therapy uses cancellous autografts to improve junctional healing. Several growth factors are undergoing clinical trials as adjuncts to this process. Utilization of recombinant human bone morphogenic proteins and other growth factors will radically alter treatment algorithms and may allow for customized tissues made from autologous cells.

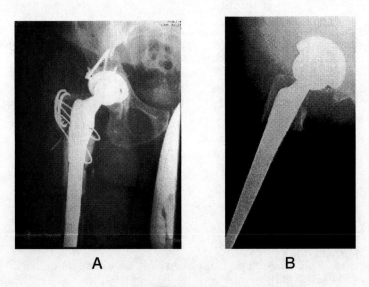

A   B

Figure 11-7

(a) pre-operative radiograph shows massive proximal femoral bone loss and two prior revision surgeries in 50-year-old man. b) intra-operative photo of transplanted femoral allograft.

Gene Therapy

Gene therapy was initially developed as a potential treatment for specific genetic disorders (adenosine deaminase deficiency, sickle cell anemia, hemophilia) and as a means of sustained systemic protein / enzyme production to cure disease. Treatment principles derived from these early studies have been applied to many disease processes including rheumatoid arthritis.

Rheumatoid arthritis is a complex disease with elements of an autoimmune process, abnormal synovial cell phenotypes, and a proliferative disorder. The role of synoviocytes in the pathophysiology of rheumatoid arthritis has been well elucidated. While debate continues over the relative primacy of T lymphocytes versus synoviocytes in explaining the pathogenesis of rheumatoid arthritis, multiple lines of evidence suggest that synoviocytes represent important, and heretofore relatively less studied targets for the development of new therapies. Semi-transformed synoviocytes produce several proteolytic enzymes associated with the tissue destruction observed in rheumatoid arthritis, including collagenase, elastase and neutral proteinases. They also express a large number of cell surface molecules that are important in the cascade of cellular and intracellular events (e.g. lymphocyte recruitment and activation) that characterize tissue inflammation. Regardless of the precise molecular events that determine the development of this semi-transformed phenotype, rheumatoid arthritis pannus synoviocytes are functionally analogous to malignant cells.

Indirect support for the pathogenic role of synoviocytes in rheumatoid arthritis, and direct support for the potential utility of therapy directed at synoviocytes can also be derived from the literature that describes the results of synovectomy. Clinical effects of surgical and medical synovectomy support the importance of synoviocytes in the pathogenesis of rheumatoid arthritis. Long-term amelioration of synovitis has also been reported following either chemical or radiation synovectomy. More recently synovectomy of the knee has been accomplished using arthroscopic procedures. These therapies have been de-emphasized in recent years because of drawbacks including cost, inability to treat large numbers of joints, and morbidity such as joint stiffness. However, the results of these trials clearly suggest the potential efficacy of therapy directed primarily at the synovium.

There is extensive literature that describes the use of gene transfer as a means to effect transgenic expression of herpes simplex thymidine kinase within a defined group of target cells. Most often the targeted cells have been neoplastic in origin; other cell types have also been used as targets for thymidine kinase gene transfer. In most animal model systems studied, and in all early human clinical trials, the transgenic expression of herpes simplex thymidine kinase has been used to convert the nucleoside analog gancyclovir into toxic phosphorylated metabolites. Phosphorylation of gancyclovir is associated with cytotoxicity through interference with DNA synthesis and alteration of other pathways of nucleotide metabolism and function.

In addition to direct cytotoxic effects in transduced cells, certain types of transduced cells can mediate a cytotoxic "bystander effect" on neighboring non-transduced cells. This bystander effect can greatly magnify the regional cytolytic effect associated with this type of gene therapy. Transgenic expression of herpes simplex thymidine kinase combined with systemic administration of gancyclovir is a molecular method for cell specific cytolysis. This plasmid DNA approach to targeted cytolysis is a potentially new approach for rheumatoid arthritis. The concept of molecular synovectomy for rheumatoid arthritis will attract other technologies in the future as its benefits are confirmed.

A Phase 1 dose escalation study of intra-articular pNGVL-TK plasmid DNA followed by systemic gancyclovir (hereafter referred to as TK/GCV) for the treatment of active rheumatoid synovitis of the knee is currently underway. This trial will study 4 doses of pNGVL-TK plasmid DNA over a dosing range of one and one-half logs. A constant dose of intravenous gancyclovir (5 mg/kg administered twice daily for three days) will be used for each dose of pNGVL-TK plasmid DNA tested. The three major goals of this Phase I trial are; 1) to establish that rheumatoid synoviocytes can be transfected in vivo using intra-articular administration of naked pNGVL-TK plasmid DNA; 2) to establish the safety of the plasmid based thymidine kinase/gancyclovir intra-articular treatment and; 3) to identify biological effects specific to the thymidine kinase/gancyclovir gene therapy.

In order to achieve these goals, arthroscopically guided synovial biopsy of the knee has been chosen for the acquisition of synovial tissues for histologic and molecular analyses. Clinical examination, combined with power Doppler sonography, represent the best non-invasive methods available to monitor the clinical effects associated with thymidine kinase/gancyclovir gene therapy over an extended period of observation. The future success of human gene therapy depends on careful safety trials, societal informed consent, strict adherence to institutional review board guidance, and a high degree of investigator ethics. Because of the high profile surrounding any gene therapy protocol, unintentional acts of omission can have disastrous results.

Considerable effort is currently underway to understand the molecular basis for orthopedic diseases, especially osteoarthritis. Many population-based studies demonstrate variations in disease incidence independent of other risk factors such as obesity. The future of molecular diagnosis and perhaps treatment depends on careful study of these genetic differences.

The future holds the promise of significant improvement in diagnosis and disease identification. Current molecular techniques will likely lead to entirely new classifications. Current methods of classification rely on descriptive terms such as "juvenile onset", "pauciarticular", or "degenerative joint disease." Classification schemes will shift to specify the precise molecular abnormalities leading to these disorders, to make intelligent predictions of a patient's future with respect to musculoskeletal diseases based on genetic profiles.

Operating Room Design

In order to utilize these advances in therapy, operating rooms in the future will be very different. With the advent of competent surgical navigation and robotics, future operating rooms will likely be highly specialized. These operating rooms will have sophisticated imaging technology and will function independently of radiologists. The issues for construction in the future will not be adequate lighting, but sufficient connectivity for web-based imaging software, adequate cooling for computers, and hands-free devices for virtual imaging. There will be micro-CT and micro-MRIs that can function similar to the current low radiation C-arm. These imaging modalities will not only allow anatomic definition, but also guide precise, minimally invasive procedures.

Impact on Patient Care and Teaching

There will be substantial changes in practice patterns. The current trend toward outpatient therapies will likely continue. Reimbursement schemes currently favor inpatient treatment and allow hospitals higher reimbursement. One of the great challenges for the future will be to revolutionize reimbursement protocols to benefit institutions and surgeons who invest time and money in new and more expensive technologies without compromising optimal patient care.

Academic medicine must anticipate these changes because they will change the needs of training programs. There will be new focus on molecular techniques necessary for diagnosis and treatment. Orthopedic surgeons will need to be facile with image interpretation and acquisition technology. Orthopedic surgeons will need to have operational familiarity with navigation systems and robotics. There will be complex issues of credentialing and considerable effort spent on training and safety. The American Academy of Orthopedic Surgeons is at the forefront of these educational changes. At the national headquarters in Chicago, there is an Orthopedic Learning Center where courses in surgical technique are conducted in a simulated operating room with hands-on teaching from experienced faculty.

Medical schools will need to change as well. The current trend favors the hiring of clinical-track faculty rather than tenure tract faculty. The concept is to promote high levels of clinical activity with no research commitment in an academic environment. Tenure track faculty have almost the same clinical demands if they want competitive salaries and there are many inducements to working with industry. This outsourcing of excellence can lead to important inventions that generate institutional royalties. But there are also incentives for young surgeons to leave institutions and academic medicine to take advantage of royalty agreements that precede their employment. The leadership of our medical schools must devise equitable incentives that promote entrepreneurial behavior and legitimate individual success.

Conclusions

The future of orthopedic surgery is one of extraordinary improvement in our ability to provide safe, high quality restoration of function. This brief overview provides only a few current trends and opportunities. We can look to the future with limitless optimism as molecular biology, tissue engineering and new technology fulfill the products of our imagination.

CHAPTER 12

PLASTIC SURGERY

WILLIAM M. KUZON, JR., M.D., PH.D.

Introduction

Plastic surgery is a specialty with a heritage of innovation, technical virtuosity, and a dedication to perfection in the surgical treatment of a vast array of physical deformities. Reconstructive surgery is the foundation that keeps Plastic Surgery at the forefront of surgical creativity, and research in Plastic Surgery is the raw material to maintain the foundation of the specialty.

"Prediction is very hard, particularly of the future" (Neils Bohr, 1885-1962). Nevertheless, there are strong indications that basic research in the areas of tissue engineering, transplantation immunology, neuroregeneration, and wound healing will interact with reconstructive surgery in the areas of craniofacial, hand, nerve, and general reconstructive surgery to substantially enhance the surgical management of patients with debilitating and disfiguring deformities. This thesis will focus on the management of major congenital anomalies of hard or soft tissue, the restoration of body parts lost or injured as a result of trauma or surgical excision, functional reconstruction of significant neuromuscular disabilities, the treatment of chronic wounds, and a possible future that includes scarless surgery. Areas within the scope of Plastic Surgical practice have been omitted not because they are unimportant, but because they are covered in other parts of this monograph.

Wound Healing

Plastic Surgery is defined as a specialty by its ability to manage problem wounds. The etiology of these wounds can include trauma, infections, degenerative diseases, and surgical insult. Chronic wounds alone are a huge health burden in the United States with costs easily reaching tens of thousands of dollars for each affected patient (1). This huge health burden is the direct result of our imperfect understanding of normal and pathologic wound healing. Recognizing this, wound healing is an area of significant research activity in Plastic Surgery and this research holds promise to significantly change the way chronic or difficult wounds are managed (2).

Wound healing is now recognized to be a complex interaction between a pro-inflammatory milieu and a milieu that supports the proliferation and differentiation of cells that enact tissue repair or regeneration (3). Chronic wounds result from an imbalance in the milieu that engenders a state of prolonged inflammation. Therapies aimed at "jump-starting" the stalled orderly progression of wound healing events have recently begun to impact patient management.

Recombinant human platelet derived growth factor (PGDF) or becaplermin has recently been shown to accelerate the healing of pressure sores (4). Other growth factors, including FGF, VEGF, and TGF are under intense investigation (5). Novel delivery systems, including "interactive dressings" that employ engineered or "designer" cells to produce growth factors within a wound may impact clinical care in the near future (Figure 1) (6). The promotion of an anti-inflammatory milieu via the use of hyperbaric oxygen, colloidal dressings, or negative pressure devices may also significantly enhance our ability to treat chronic wounds.

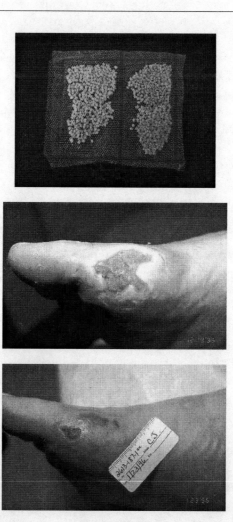

Figure 12-1

a) Interactive wound dressing composed of keratinocytes bonded to sephadex beads and incased in a permeable membrane. b) Diabetic foot ulcer – pre treatment. c) After

The most significant new therapies for chronic wounds will come from research to clarify the basic biology of wounds. Gene chip technology is now being actively exploited in this area, with protein-chip technology soon to follow (7). Understanding the genomic and proteomic responses to wounding will lead to a revolution in the management of problem wounds. Instead of pursuing growth factors or inflammatory mediators one by one, these new technologies permit recognization of patterns of synergistic expression so that one can utilize multiple, simultaneous factors to optimize the wound environment. New cellular, pharmacological, and physical therapies should significantly enhance the ability to treat this fundamental surgical problem.

Scars

Because skin heals via reparative rather than regenerative processes, wounds result in scars in post-natal mammals. More than an aesthetic concern, scars result in substantial morbidity. The scarring associated with burns or other traumatic injures can limit growth, impair joint motion, limit tendon gliding, and result in dysfunction of critical oral or ocular sphincters. The scarring that results from cleft palate repair significantly impedes maxillary growth, necessitating major skeletal surgery in afflicted patients (8). Pathologic scarring (hypertrophic scars and keloids) represent a significant problem for susceptible patients after burns or other injuries (Figure 2). Surgical scar release, steroid injections, silicone sheet application, low-energy radiotherapy, and pressure dressings are the current mainstay of therapy for disabling scars. These therapies are both crude and empiric. Because scars represent a major area of concern for Plastic Surgeons, scarless healing will be a major objective for the specialty in the next century.

Like chronic wounds, problem scars are the result of an imbalance between competing milieus. Collagen deposition, angiogenesis, and cellular proliferation must give way to collagen degradation and collagen remodeling and a reduction in cellularity during the scar remodeling phase of scarring. Recent data indicate that differential expression of TGF-b isoforms are observed in pathologic compared with normal scars. Keloids and hypertrophic scars were found have diminished expression of TGF-b3 and increased expression of TGF-b1 when compared with non-pathologic scars (9). In addition, the observation, during the first trimester, that fetal skin heals via a scarless, regenerative process has helped to define the factors that engender scars in adult animals (10). These observations, combined with contemporary gene and protein chip technology will point the way towards a rational, non-empiric approach to problem scars in the next century. The scarring process represents the major limitation in the ability to perform reconstruction of may critical body parts, particularly those with delicate anatomy such as the ear or eyelid. If scarring can be controlled or eliminated, a renaissance will occur in reconstructive surgery that will rival the advances resulting from the development of microvascular free tissue transfer and myocutaneous flaps.

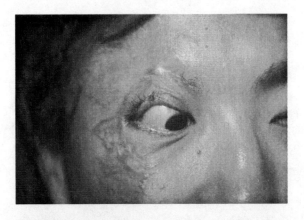

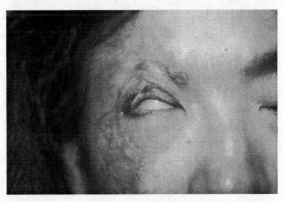

Figure 12-2

Hypertrophic scar with contracture producing symptomatic lagopthalmos. The scar resulted from an abrasion during a motor vehicle accident; there was no significant tissue loss. The potential serious sequelae of scars can include blindness from exposure keratitis as in this patient.

Flap Surgery and Composite Tissue Reconstruction

Microvascular technique and advances in the understanding of the blood supply to composite tissues (the angiosome concept) have revolutionized reconstructive surgery. This anatomical knowledge and technical ability free the reconstructive surgeon to harvest tissue from distant sites and provide for complex, composite tissue requirements in the recipient site. Reconstructive options are limited by the expandability and by the anatomy of donor sites. For example, although one can reconstruct complex oromandibular defects with the free fibula flap, the results are far from aesthetically or functionally perfect and come at the expense of significant morbidity in the donor site (Figure 3). In addition, microvascular thrombosis or gradient ischemia sometimes results in tissue necrosis, with catastrophic results for the patient (11). Research holds the promise for an improved future in the area of flap surgery.

Ischemia reperfusion injury is a complex pathophysiologic process. Tissue injury in this setting is the result of neutrophil-mediated oxygen-free radical damage to cell membranes. Neutrophil adhesion and chemotaxis are the initiating events in

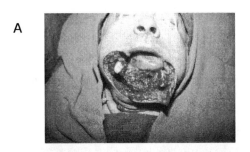

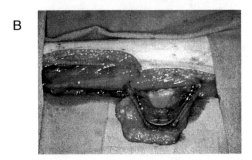

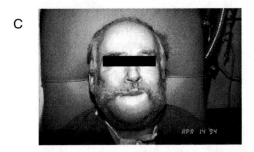

Figure 12-3
A) Oromandibular defect after composite resection of squamous cell carcinoma. B) Fibula osteoseptocutaneous flap, in situ, after osteotomy. C) Completed reconstruction. The fibula free flap was combined with a radial forearm free flap that was used to reconstruct the chin and lower lip.

ischemia-reperfusion injury (12). Blocking CD18 and other receptors responsible for neutrophil adhesion in injured tissue represents one rational investigative strategy to ameliorate tissue damage after ischemia and reperfusion. Ischemic pre-conditioning of tissue prior to flap strategy has been a focus of research in flap surgery. These studies indicate that adenosine receptors may be a target for pharmacological agents intended to reduce ischemic tissue injury, and may become a therapeutic modality used prior to free tissue transfer (13).

Even if surgeons overcome ischemia-reperfusion injury, microvascular thrombosis, and other factors that result in flap failure, they will still be limited by available autogenous donor tissue when attempting to reconstruct complex tissue deformities. Two areas of current research, composite tissue transplantation and tissue engineering, may release the reconstructive surgeon from the bonds of available autogenous anatomy spawn a renaissance in reconstructive surgery.

The field of composite tissue transplantation was electrified in 1998 and 1999 when several groups performed allogeneic hand transplants to reconstruct patients with previous upper extremity amputations (14). Although the results of these procedures have been disappointing, advances in our understanding of transplantation biology may open the door to the use of allogeneic tissue for the reconstruction of complex deformities. Unlike solid organ transplantation, where the use of immunosuppressive pharmacological agents has led to organ transplantation becoming accepted in the mainstream of surgical therapies, the transplantation of limbs or other composite tissues remains on the fringe of acceptable clinical practice. It is generally agreed that the negative long-term consequences of immunosuppressive therapy preclude the use of these agents for problems that are not life threatening. As a consequence, research in this area has focused on the induction of tissue-specific tolerance (15). If surgeons can induce tolerance to complex tissues without general immunosuppression, composite tissue transplantation may become a reality.

Two lines of research hold promise in this area. The first is the use of monoclonal antibodies or other pharmacologic agents that selectively inhibit rejection of allogenic tissue without impairing host response to pathogens or to tumors. MR-1, an anti-CD40 ligand monoclonal antibody, has been shown to allow transplantation of rat hindlimbs and peripheral nerves across major histocompatibility barriers without a rejection response (16). The ability to ameliorate peripheral nerve rejection is particularly significant because, unlike many other tissues, Schwann cells trigger both a TH1 and a TH2 response by the host immune system. Whether true tolerance is induced via MR-1 administration remains a source of controversy. Nevertheless, this line of research holds significant promise.

The second strategy being studied in this area is the induction of an immunologic chimeric state in the recipient animal by manipulation of the immune system prior to transplantation of allogeneic composite tissues. Using miniature swine, Lee et al. have induced mixed chimerism in a large animal model and have demonstrated that prolonged survival of transplanted composite tissues is possible without immunosuppressive agents (17). Although significant hurdles remain, the clinical application of composite tissue transplantation is poised for a major explosion in the foreseeable future.

Tissue Engineering

Tissue engineering represents a novel strategy for the replacement of damaged or missing tissues, and it holds promise for all fields of surgery (18). Plastic Surgery has fully embraced the potential of tissue engineering to impact reconstructive surgery and, in fact, the innovators in this field used ear reconstruction as their "proof of concept" (19).

The basic concept of tissue engineering is to expand the component cells of a given tissue and then to assemble them into a functioning tissue. Tissue that is newly-generated by this method can be constructed for specific reconstructive needs and

A
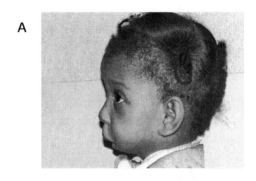

B
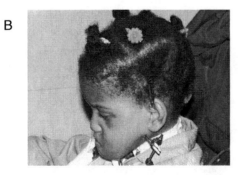

Figure 12-4
Distraction osteogenesis. A) Preoperative photograph demonstrating micrognathia requiring a tracheostomy. B) After mandibular distraction; note the bi-planar distractor.

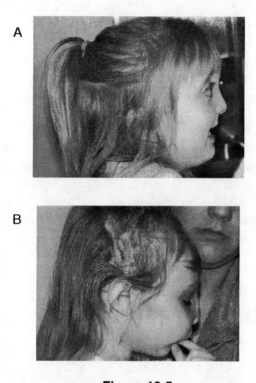

Figure 12-5

Distraction osteogenesis. A) Child with syndromic craniosynostoses and midface hypoplasia. B) After distraction osteogenesis of the midface.

is therefore potentially of immense versatility in reconstructive surgery. One form of endogenous tissue engineering, distraction osteogenesis is already widely applied for the correction of craniofacial anomalies (20).

Mandibular distraction osteogenesis has become a mainstay of therapy for patients with hemifacial microsomia, congenital micrognathia, and acquired mandibular deformities (Figure 4). This same technique is now under investigation for the correction of major midfacial and cranial deformities (Figure 5). The future is likely to see a significant expansion of the use of distraction osteogenesis in craniofacial surgery, and the age of the major, open craniofacial osteotomy may be closing.

In addition to the use of bone distraction, tissue engineering is poised to revolutionize reconstructive surgery. Skin or dermis substitutes can be considered first-generation tissue engineered products. A second generation of products is likely to encompass structural tissues, and in particular cartilage. The avascular nature of hyaline cartilage makes it an ideal target for research in tissue engineering because there is no requirement to generate a new vascular supply for the engineered tissue. Ear, nose, and joint reconstruction may be significantly enhanced by the ability of the tissue engineer to combine an alloplastic, biodegradable matrix with chondrocytes expanded from a small biopsy of autologous tissue (19). As the basic interaction between cells and stromal matrix is understood, and as understanding of neoangiogensis improves, control of cellular behavior should allow the generation of increasingly more complex tissues for use in reconstruction.

Craniofacial Surgery

Technology allowing distraction of the craniofacial skeleton and the potential of tissue engineering may significantly impact craniofacial surgery in the next 100 years. An understanding of craniofacial developmental biology may lead to major advances in the diagnosis and treatment of syndromic and non-syndromic craniosynostosis and of facial clefting.

It is now known that syndromic craniosynostosis is the result of mutations in the FGF receptor (21). In addition, it is now clear that the dura mater controls the patency of cranial sutures in the developing skull (22). Cranial vault reshaping and osteotomies to reposition the bones of the craniofacial skeleton may be unnecessary if therapeutic agents to directly control cranial suture biology can be found.

The treatment of facial clefting, including the treatment of cleft lip and palate, has changed little in over 30 years. Soft tissue defects are repaired via local tissue rearrangements or by augmentation with distant tissue. Bony clefts are left unrepaired or are closed using bone grafts. Lack of progress in this area likely relates to our poor understanding of the causes of facial clefts. Recently, a unified theory of embryologic dysgenesis that may explain both craniosysnosis and clefting has been proposed (23). By mapping the developing forebrain via specific genetic markers, an improved concept of facial embryogenesis has resulted in the concept that facial clefts are due to deletions in specific zones of the neurotube and craniosynostoses are due to failure of differentiation between adjacent zones. This concept requires further study, but may revolutionize the manner in which surgeons approach congenital facial deformities. No breakthroughs in the management of craniofacial deformities will be forthcoming until the etiology is further defined.

Neuromuscular Reconstruction

Traumatic injuries, surgical extirpations, and congenital anomalies can result in significant physical disability in afflicted patients. Despite advances in microneural surgery and in muscle transfers to restore lost joint motion or facial animation, patients with significant neuromuscular injuries are often left with significant, life-long disabilities. In the next century, advances in this area, fueled by basic research, promise to improve the results of peripheral nerve repairs, to preserve target organs from atrophy, and even to generate, de novo, functional skeletal muscle.

Three challenges confront the patient with a nerve injury. The first is to guide and support axons as they regenerate across a nerve repair and elongate to reach the target, denervated tissue. The second is to have sufficiently preserved target tissue to allow for reinnervation. The third is to re-establish functional circuitry with appropriate neural pathways. All three of these processes can be impaired and result in sub-optimal recovery; all three of these processes are the subject of intense research that may result in a significant improvement in the treatment of patients with nerve injuries or muscle injury.

When a peripheral nerve is cut, the proximal axonal stumps will begin to elongate, sending out regenerating units that, if supported properly, will reach target motor or sensory end-organs, form new synapses, and allow resumption of function. In order to elongate, axons require trophic support from Schwann cells and an appropriate, endoneurial environment. Schwann cells provide trophic support to axons and, through specific cell-cell interactions, guide axons as they elongate. An appropriate endoneurial environment consists of longitudinal, basement membrane lined tubes that provide structure and restrict axonal elongation to the appropriate direction. If an end-to-end nerve coaptation is possible, the distal nerve stump is the best available environment. Even under these circumstances, however, the slow rate of axonal elongation and a reduced number of axons eventually form functional synapses result in impaired recovery. Nerve growth factor was the first of a number of neurotrophic growth factors that have been shown to speed axonal elongation and to improve reinnervation of target muscles or sensory organs (24). Delivery systems allowing the use of neurotrophic growth factors in the clinical setting remain investigational. In the future, transient up regulation of the expression of neurotrophic factors may be possible via viral vectors (25), and the use of neurotrophic pharmaceuticals such as FK506 may become commonplace (26). If surgeons can improve the speed of axonal regeneration, they will significantly impact recovery, because denervation time is a significant determinant of recovery for denervated-reinnervated skeletal muscle (27).

Sensory receptors appear to remain receptive to reinnervation many years after axotomy while skeletal muscle undergoes a process of denervation atrophy that results in a resistance to reinnervation within 18 months. Even if axons reach a muscle target, "denervation atrophy" often prevents appreciable recovery of function. As a result, preservation of skeletal muscle during denervation is under active investigation. Several strategies have been studied; the most promising are sensory-preservation, motor babysitting, and electrical stimulation. Sensory preservation involves directing an expendable sensory nerve into a target to maintain the intramuscular endoneurial sheaths and to allow factors elaborated by sensory axons to trophically support the muscle fibers (28). This strategy may allow reinnervation of the intrinsic muscles of the hand in high ulnar nerve lesions if the median nerve is intact in the same patient.

Motor-motor babysitting involves directing non-specific motor axons to the target muscles to allow for rapid muscle reinnervation. These axons "baby-sit" the target muscle while motion specific axons regenerate from a distant source to reach the muscle. The non-specific reinnervation is then replaced by motion-specific axons. Although two episodes of denervation and reinnervation are required, this approach has become common for patients with facial paralysis and may be useful for patients with other peripheral nerve lesions (29).

In addition to these surgical strategies, electrical stimulation represents a direct attempt to preserve denervated skeletal muscle for long periods. With appropriate stimulation parameters, it is possible to preserve skeletal muscle mass and force capacity for many months (30). Although subsequent recovery after nerve regeneration was not improved in some experimental studies and although clinical trials of electrical stimulation have been difficult to interpret, it seems clear that further research in this area will occur and may result in significant benefit for patients with nerve injuries.

In order to direct axons back to denervated tissue, an appropriate environment must support axonal elongation. Although the distal stump of the severed nerve is the best available regeneration corridor, traumatic injuries and tumor resections often result in a nerve gap. In these circumstances, autologous nerve grafts are the preferred method of reconstructing nerve gaps and the resulting recovery, while poorer than for end-to-end nerve coaptation, is acceptable in many patients. There is a limited supply of expendable cutaneous sensory nerves suitable for harvest to use as grafts and the donor morbidity from harvest of these nerves ranges from a nuisance to a disabling sensory neuroma. As a consequence, the need for an "off the shelf" substitute for autologous nerve grafts is indisputable. Both tissue engineered nerve substitutes and nerve allografting have been actively studied.

Nerve conduits can be considered first generation tissue engineered nerve graft substitutes. Polyglycolic acid tubes, autologous vein conduits, and freeze-thawed muscles are used clinically, although the indications are restricted to short gaps in digital nerves. Second generation tissue engineered nerve grafts have been studied and include conduits seeded with Schwann cells, acellularized nerve or muscle matrix modified with growth factors or seeded with Schwann cells, and synthetic biomaterials with defined structures (31). It is likely that research in this area will remain a major focus and will result in tissue-engineered nerve grafts suitable for clinical use in the future.

Like composite tissue transplantation, nerve allografting is a controversial area. Nevertheless, phase I clinical trials are under way and have demonstrated remarkable recovery in patients with otherwise catastrophic brachial plexus or sciatic nerve injuries (32). Unlike hand transplants, which would require immune modulation on a permanent basis to be clinically useful, nerve allografts become fully replaced with host tissue, and therefore only temporary immunosuppression is needed. IAs host axons regenerate across a nerve allograft, the donor Schwann cells within the graft are replaced by host Schwann cells. In animal studies, no donor cells are detected at late time points (33). The most commonly used immunosuppressive agents, cyclosporine-A and FK506 are also neurotropic agents. The strategy of nerve allotransplantation is likely to find more indications in the next century.

Tissue engineering holds promise to generate new skeletal muscles to allow reconstruction of facial animation or even limb motion. Three-dimensional, self assembled skeletal muscle constructs, termed myooids, have been generated in vitro (34). These constructs are composed of stable, longitudinally oriented muscle fibers in a stromal matrix, are stable in culture for several months, and can produce measurable longitudinal force (Figure 6). Although myooids and other strategies to generate functional skeletal muscle for clinical implantation have many obstacles to surmount before becoming a clinical reality, the potential of tissue engineering to impact affected patients is enormous and makes it clear that research in this area will continue. Success in this area would represent the ultimate in surgical reconstructions: provision of an engineered, contractile tissue that would come under volitional control via synaptic communication with the patient's nervous system.

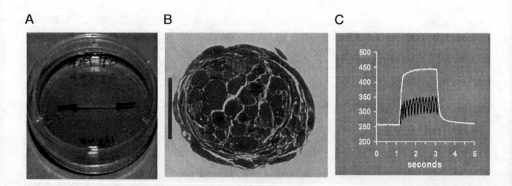

Figure 12-6

Tissue engineered skeletal muscle. A) Myooid, in vitro. B) H & E cross section of a typical myooid (bar = 100 microns). C) Force trace of a typical myooid at 6 Hz (red line) and 30 Hz (yellow line) stimulation frequency. Photographs and data courtesy of Drs. Robert Dennis and Marlene Calderon.

Summary

Plastic and Reconstructive Surgery is already an enormously diverse field focused on the fundamental problems facing all surgeons. The future of Plastic Surgery will depend on the ability to understand basic mechanisms of wound healing and scarring and on the development of new strategies to replace missing or damaged tissues. This is a broad challenge, and will require a continuation of the creative and inquisitive sprit intrinsic to the specialty. Plastic Surgeons are well equipped to meet the challenge of the next century, and patients will be the beneficiaries of therapies currently under study and of those not yet conceived.

REFERENCES

1. Schonfeld WH. Villa KF. Fastenau JM. Mazonson PD. Falanga V. An economic assessment of Apligraf (Graftskin) for the treatment of hard-to-heal venous leg ulcers. Wound Repair Regeneration. 8(4):251-7, 2000.

2. Gosain AK. What's new in plastic surgery. Journal of the American College of Surgeons. 192(3):356-65, 2001.

3. Harding KG. Morris HL. Patel GK. Science, medicine and the future: healing chronic wounds. BMJ. 324(7330):160-3, 2002.

4. Rees RS. Robson MC. Smiell JM. Perry BH. Becaplermin gel in the treatment of pressure ulcers: a phase II randomized, double-blind, placebo-controlled study. Wound Repair Regeneration. 7(3):141-7, 1999.

5. Rumalla VK. Borah GL. Cytokines, growth factors, and plastic surgery. Plastic & Reconstructive Surgery. 108(3):719-33, 2001.

6. Rees RS. Adamson BF. Lindblad WJ. Use of a cell-based interactive wound dressing to enhance healing of excisional wounds in nude mice. Wound Repair Regeneration. 9(4):297-304, 2001.

7. Cole J. Tsou R. Wallace K. Gibran N. Isik F. Comparison of normal human skin gene expression using cDNA microarrays. Wound Repair Regeneration. 9(2):77-85, 2001.

8. Peltomaki T. Vendittelli BL. Grayson BH. Cutting CB. Brecht LE. Associations between severity of clefting and maxillary growth in patients with unilateral cleft lip and palate treated with infant orthopedics. Cleft Palate-Craniofacial Journal. 38(6):582-6, 2001.

9. Chin GS. Liu W. Peled Z. Lee TY. Steinbrech DS. Hsu M. Longaker MT. Differential expression of transforming growth factor-beta receptors I and II and activation of Smad 3 in keloid fibroblasts. Plastic & Reconstructive Surgery. 108(2):423-9, 2001.

10. Longaker MT. Peled ZM. Chang J. Krummel TM. Fetal wound healing: progress report and future directions. Surgery. 130(5):785-7, 2001.

11. Khouri RK. Cooley BC. Kunselman AR. Landis JR. Yeramian P. Ingram D. Natarajan N. Benes CO. Wallemark C. A prospective study of microvascular free-flap surgery and outcome. Plastic & Reconstructive Surgery. 102(3):711-21, 1998.

12. Zamboni WA. Stephenson LL. Roth AC. Suchy H. Russell RC. Ischemia-reperfusion injury in skeletal muscle: CD 18-dependent neutrophil-endothelial adhesion and arteriolar vasoconstriction. Plastic & Reconstructive Surgery. 99(7):2002-7.

13. Pang CY. Neligan P. Zhong A. He W. Xu H. Forrest CR. Effector mechanism of adenosine in acute ischemic preconditioning of skeletal muscle against infarction. American Journal of Physiology. 273(3 Pt 2):R887-95, 1997.

14. Francois CG. Breidenbach WC. Maldonado C. Kakoulidis TP. Hodges A. Dubernard JM. Owen E. Pei G. Ren X. Barker JH. Hand transplantation: comparisons and observations of the first four clinical cases. Microsurgery. 20(8):360-71, 2000.

15. Kann BR. Furnas DW. Hewitt CW. Past, present, and future research in the field of composite tissue allotransplantation. Microsurgery. 20(8):393-9, 2000.

16. JM Rovak, DK Bishop, SY Chan, WM Kuzon, JA Faulkner, PS Cederna Short-term CD40L Monoclonal Antibody Treatment Induces Tolerance to Peripheral Nerve Allografts. Proceedings of the Plastic Surgery Research Council, 2002.

17. Bourget JL. Mathes DW. Nielsen GP. Randolph MA. Tanabe YN. Ferrara VR. Wu A. Arn S. Sachs DH. Lee WP. Tolerance to musculoskeletal allografts with transient lymphocyte chimerism in miniature swine. Transplantation. 71(7):851-6, 2001.

18. Lorenz HP. Hedrick MH. Chang J. Mehrara BJ. Longaker MT. The impact of biomolecular medicine and tissue engineering on plastic surgery in the 21st century. Plastic & Reconstructive Surgery. 105(7):2467-81, 2000.

19. Cao Y. Vacanti JP. Paige KT. Upton J. Vacanti CA. Transplantation of chondrocytes utilizing a polymer-cell construct to produce tissue-engineered cartilage in the shape of a human ear. Plastic & Reconstructive Surgery. 100(2):297-302; discussion 303-4, 1997.

20. McCarthy JG. Stelnicki EJ. Mehrara BJ. Longaker MT. Distraction osteogenesis of the craniofacial skeleton. Plastic & Reconstructive Surgery. 107(7):1812-27, 2001.

21. Morriss-Kay GM. Iseki S. Johnson D. Genetic control of the cell proliferation-differentiation balance in the developing skull vault: roles of fibroblast growth factor receptor signalling pathways. Novartis Foundation Symposium. 232:102-16, 2001.

22. Greenwald JA. Mehrara BJ. Spector JA. Warren SM. Crisera FE. Fagenholz PJ. Bouletreau PJ. Longaker MT. Regional differentiation of cranial suture-associated dura mater in vivo and in vitro: implications for suture fusion and patency. Journal of Bone & Mineral Research. 15(12):2413-30, 2000.

23. William Y. Hoffman, M.D., Personal Communication, 2002.

24. Frostick SP. Yin Q. Kemp GJ. Schwann cells, neurotrophic factors, and peripheral nerve regeneration. Microsurgery. 18(7):397-405, 1998.

25. Tepper OM. Mehrara BJ. Gene therapy in plastic surgery. Plastic & Reconstructive Surgery. 109(2):716-34, 2002.

26. Navarro X. Udina E. Ceballos D. Gold BG. Effects of FK506 on nerve regeneration and reinnervation after graft or tube repair of long nerve gaps. Muscle & Nerve. 24(7):905-15, 2001.

27. Kobayashi J. Mackinnon SE. Watanabe O. Ball DJ. Gu XM. Hunter DA. Kuzon WM Jr. The effect of duration of muscle denervation on functional recovery in the rat model. Muscle & Nerve. 20(7):858-66, 1997.

28. Bain JR. Veltri KL. Chamberlain D. Fahnestock M. Improved functional recovery of denervated skeletal muscle after temporary sensory nerve innervation. Neuroscience. 103(2):503-10, 2001.

29. Mersa B. Tiangco DA. Terzis JK. Efficacy of the "baby-sitter" procedure after prolonged denervation. Journal of Reconstructive Microsurgery. 16(1):27-35, 2000.

30. Nicolaidis SC. Williams HB. Muscle preservation using an implantable electrical system after nerve injury and repair. Microsurgery. 21(6):241-7, 2001.

31. Mohammad JA. Warnke PH. Pan YC. Shenaq S. Increased axonal regeneration through a biodegradable amnionic tube nerve conduit: effect of local delivery and incorporation of nerve growth factor/hyaluronic acid media. Annals of Plastic Surgery. 44(1):59-64, 2000.

32. Mackinnon SE. Doolabh VB. Novak CB. Trulock EP. Clinical outcome following nerve allograft transplantation. Plastic & Reconstructive Surgery. 107(6):1419-29, 2001.

33. Midha R. Mackinnon SE. Becker LE. The fate of Schwann cells in peripheral nerve allografts. Journal of Neuropathology & Experimental Neurology. 53(3):316-22, 1994.

34. Dennis RG. Kosnik PE 2nd. Excitability and isometric contractile properties of mammalian skeletal muscle constructs engineered in vitro. In Vitro Cellular & Developmental Biology. Animal. 36(5):327-35, 2000.

CHAPTER 13

BREAST SURGERY

ALFRED E. CHANG, M.D., EDWIN G. WILKINS, M.D., MICHAEL S. SABEL, M.D.

20th Century Paradigms for the Surgical Management of Breast Cancer

The surgical management for breast cancer has witnessed dramatic changes during the 20th century. At the beginning of the 20th century, Halsted created a new paradigm in the surgical management of breast cancer that became the mainstay of therapy for the first 50 years of that century. Halsted hypothesized that breast cancer had an orderly natural progression that started from the primary tumor that progressed to the regional lymph nodes; and, eventually to distant sites beyond. Standard therapy involved the radical resection of the primary tumor and en bloc resection of the regional nodes.(Figure 1) (1) In the second half of the 20th century, a new paradigm emerged based upon the concept that breast cancer did not follow this predictable, orderly progression. Instead, breast cancer was postulated to be a systemic cancer from the outset, and that the involvement of lymph nodes was merely an epiphenomenon reflecting the fact that the risk of visceral involvement paralleled nodal involvement. This concept was championed by Umberto Veronesi and Bernard Fisher who pioneered these concepts through seminal randomized trials involving different approaches to the surgical management of nodal tissues as well as the primary tumor.(2-4) These trials paved the way to our current viewpoints regarding the treatment of breast cancers and their biological behaviors.

Today, the surgical aspects regarding breast care treatment involve three different areas: treatment of the primary tumor, staging of the axillary lymph nodes, and reconstruction of the patient requiring mastectomy. Several major advances in the adjuvant treatment of breast cancer have dramatically affected breast cancer surgery. These include the role of radiation therapy in reducing local recurrence after wide excision of primary breast tumor and the discovery that hormonal manipulation and systemic cytotoxic drugs can eradicate residual micrometastatic disease in women and prolong survival after surgical therapy. With respect to the primary tumor, it is incumbent on the surgeon to determine whether or not the patient is a breast-sparing candidate. This requires assessment of whether the tumor is unifocal or multifocal; and, if the lesion can be removed with negative margins so that adjuvant radiation therapy can be administered. As far as the axillary nodes, it is incumbent on the surgeon to assess the nodal status of the patient for prognostic information in order to guide subsequent systemic therapy. In the case of breast reconstruction, it is a matter of quality of life. The new century will see dramatic paradigm shifts in the treatment

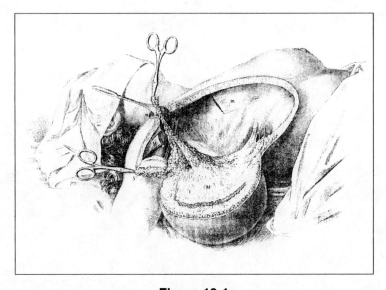

Figure 13-1
Drawing of radical mastectomy from Halsted's original report (Reprinted from Ann Surg 20: 497, 1894).

of breast cancer just as great as has been witnessed by the last century. The main reason for this will be due to new insights regarding the biology of breast cancer and its progression at the molecular level.

Unlocking the Human Genome and Its Implications to Cancer Treatment

One of the restrictions scientists and clinicians were faced with in the 20th century was defining cancers at the macroscopic and whole cell level. This was reflective of what tools were available to clinicians and dictated how we approached treatment of a spectrum of diseases. Cancers were looked upon as a spontaneously arising disease due to either environmental or genetic predilections that resulted in disorderly proliferation of cells that can spread to other organs. Little was known regarding the mechanisms for genesis or subsequent propagation of cancer cells at the subcellular level. A new era was ushered in when the human genome was mapped and reported in February, 2001 by Francis Collins and Craig Venter.(5, 6) With a map of the genome, a door was opened to define the genetic differences that are present in diseased conditions, particularly cancers.(7, 8) Cancers are now thought of as genetic diseases. The overall behavior of a cancer must be determined by the expression of the genes within it. There is currently an explosion of studies in laboratories throughout the world to apply molecular tools to characterize the genetic abnormalities that are associated with specific cancers. By identifying unique differences in gene expression, one can determine the biological behavior of tumors and target important cell signaling or metastatic mechanisms involved in the progression of the cancer. Two of the more important molecular tools that basic scientists are employing are microarray and proteomic assays.

How Molecular Approaches have Impacted on Breast Cancer Knowledge

Microarray technology provides a method for monitoring the RNA expression levels of many thousands of genes simultaneously in primary tumors and cell lines. A microarray is an orderly arrangement of known or unknown DNA samples attached to a solid support. Using these support systems, the expression of thousands of genes in a cancer can be compared to a normal complement of genes and differences identified.(Figure 2) Variation in gene dosage through either amplification or deletion of genomic regions is a frequent feature of human cancer. Amplification of

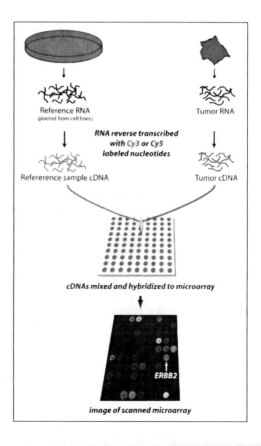

Figure 13-2

Schematic diagram of cDNA microarray analysis of tumor samples. (Reprinted with permission from Molecular Intervention 2: 103, 2002).

genomic regions is believed to result in the overexpression of genes that drive cancer development and/or are involved in conferring drug resistance. Amplification events in breast cancer have attracted particular attention because they can often be used as clinical markers of tumor behavior such as Her2/neu.

In theory, it should be possible to identify sets of genes whose expression or lack of expression defines each individual property of a cancer, including its precise diagnosis and clinical behavior. Sorlie et al. recently reported upon 85 cDNA microarray experiments representing 78 breast cancers, three fibroadenomas, and four normal breast tissues which were analyzed by hierarchical clustering.(9) Among the specimens, there was considerable variation in the pattern of gene expression among the tumors. This variation was partly due to changes in the levels of certain cell types within the tumors, such as endothelial cells, stromal cells, adipose-enriched normal breast cells, B and T lymphocytes and macrophages. Once genes characteristic of these cell types had been excluded, the authors selected a subset of 456 genes, called "intrinsic genes" that still showed considerable variation in expression levels between different tumors. Using hierarchical clustering methods, the 78 carcinomas and 7 nonmalignant breast samples were analyzed.(Figure 3) Five tumor subgroups

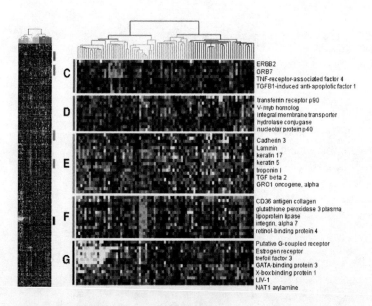

Figure 13-3

Gene expression patterns of 85 samples representing 78 breast cancers, 3 benign tumors, 4 normal tissues analyzed by hierarchical clustering. Color bars represent inserts presented in C-G: (C) ERBB2 amplicon cluster; (D) novel unknown cluster; (E) basal epithelial cell-enriched cluster; (F) normal breast-like cluster; and (G) luminal epithelial gene cluster containing ER (Reprinted with permission from PNAS 98: 10871, 2001).

were identified according to genetic clustering. These included a basal-epithelial-like group, ERBB2-overexpressing group, normal breast-like group, and a luminal epithelial/estrogen receptor positive group that could be divided into at least two subgroups with distinctive expression profiles. Survival analysis on a subcohort of patients with locally advanced cancer uniformly treated in a prospective study showed significantly different outcomes for the patients belonging to the various groups. These findings substantiate the validity of genetic profiling as a means to classify breast cancers other than just by grade or size which represent the conventional histological staging criteria used today.

Another group recently reported the use of microarray analysis to identify high risk breast cancer patients in earlier staged breast cancers. Van't Veer and co-workers evaluated primary breast tumors from 117 young (<55 years) patients, and applied a supervised classification method to identify a gene expression signature strongly predictive of a short interval to distant metastases.(10) All these patients were node negative to begin with. The poor prognosis signature consisted of genes regulating cell cycle, invasion, metastasis and angiogenesis. The "poor prognosis" signature out performed all currently used clinical parameters in predicting disease outcome. Based on their analysis, the authors concluded that many patients who might routinely be recommended to undergo adjuvant systemic therapy based on consensus recommendations could be spared the treatment based on molecular profiling. These findings clearly herald the future obsolescence of lymph node staging.

Recently, using microarray analysis, distinct genetic differences have been found between primary tumors from patients with hereditary breast cancer compared to sporadic cancers.(11) This would indicate that the pathogenesis of their development are clearly different. Furthermore, this can be one method to identify BRCA1 or 2 carriers. Another report by Unger et al. utilized microarray analysis to distinguish whether or not multicentric breast tumors arose from the same tumor clone.(12) This technique allows for a useful diagnostic tool for determining tumor clonality and heterogeneity that would have impact on therapeutic decisions in patients with multiple breast tumors.

As a complementary analysis, proteomics is the elucidation of all of the proteins encoded for by the genome. Information generated by microarray analysis does not provide the functional status of the cell regarding the abundance, activity, post-translational modifications, and localization of the corresponding proteins. Unlike the genome, which is a relatively stable information archive, each cell type has its own unique proteome, and within that subset, each cell type has a changing proteome in response not only to the progression of the malignancy but also to therapy and environmental factors.(13) An important tool employed with proteomic technology is laser capture microdissection (LCM). LCM technology allows investigators to isolate selected cells out of a stained tissue section. LCM takes advantage of an infrared laser that melts a thermo-sensitive ethylene vinyl acetate polymer film over selected single cells. This thermoplastic film forms a solid composite with the tissue at the targeted sites. The film holding the captured cells is then lifted from the remaining tissue section, and cells can be analyzed for DNA, RNA, and protein content. Two-dimensional gel electrophoresis is still the mainstay of most proteomic analysis. New, exciting approaches of multiparameter protein characterization are being developed.(13) Proteomic research will also result in new molecular classification of tumors, new molecular targets for therapy, biomarkers for early detection, and new endpoints for therapeutic efficacy and toxicity.

21st Century Paradigms for the Surgical Management of Breast Cancer

The genomic revolution will have dramatic impact on how clinicians will treat breast cancer. One significant impact will be how we stage cancers. It is predicted that the current staging system that employs tumor size, nodal status and evidence of metastatic disease will become obsolete. There will be a new classification of breast tumors based upon the genetic expression or profile of individual tumors. As noted above, the genetic profile of tumors will predict which tumors will have a poor prognosis. It is also anticipated that new molecular targets will be identified through microarray and proteomic research for which therapeutic modalities can be tailored.

The necessity to stage the axillary lymph nodes will no longer exist when more precise prognostic genetic markers are identified. Surgeons will no longer perform axillary node dissections or sentinel lymph node biopsies in the future. Rather, the focus of the surgeon will be concentrated in the management of the primary tumor and attempts to achieve local control. In this regard, the application of neoadjuvant systemic therapy to reduce the size of the primary tumor will become a standard approach. The topics of new primary treatment modalities and neoadjuvant systemic options are reviewed in the next two sections.

Treatment of the Primary Tumor
In Situ Ablation Therapies

Along with a new paradigm in the surgical treatment of breast cancer and a new understanding of the natural biology of the disease, advances in technology have also helped shift the approach to early-stage breast cancer towards less invasive modalities. The technology for stereotactic guided localization of non-palpable breast tumors was introduced in 1986, and is now available in virtually all communities for biopsy of these lesions. Similarly, advances in ultrasound and magnetic resonance imaging (MRI) technology has markedly improved our ability to visualize and biopsy breast tumors.

The goals of breast cancer surgery have always been local tumor control and survival, and more recently have included satisfactory cosmetic results. These goals have been increasingly well met with improvement in breast imaging techniques and the increased detection of smaller cancers, improved techniques for breast irradiation, and more effective systemic cytotoxic and hormonal therapies. As the pendulum continues to swing towards breast-sparing therapy, there is increasing interest in further meeting these goals without surgery. As the technology improves, it is becoming more feasible to treat early-stage breast tumors without excision and its attendant scar. Several methods have been described to ablate all the tissue around the tumor while leaving the remaining breast unaltered.(14, 15)

Radiofrequency Ablation

Radiofrequency ablation (RFA) destroys tumors by heat, although the heat is not conducted directly. Rather, an electrical current alternating at a frequency of approximately 400 kHz causes intracellular ions in the tissues to vibrate in response and create frictional heating. A probe connected to a generator is placed by ultrasound guidance into the tumor. Once in position, the prongs are deployed to evenly distribute the current. The temperature at the site of the tumor is raised to 95 degrees Celcius and maintained for about 15 minutes.

While significant experience has been obtained with RFA for the ablation of liver tumors (16, 17), it is increasingly being used for other tumors.(18-21) Preclinical animal trials have demonstrated the feasibility of utilizing this technology in the treatment of breast cancer.(22, 23) Jeffery et al described their results in five women who underwent radiofrequency ablation prior to surgical resection in a feasibility study.(24) The average tumor size was 4 to 7cm, and only a portion of the tumor was treated so the margin between ablated and nonablated tissue could be assessed. Viability stains of the ablated tissue showed complete cell death in four of the five patients. Izzo et al reported the results of a pilot trial of RFA in 26 patients with T1 and T2 breast cancers.(25) They achieved complete coagulation necrosis in 25 of the patients. Singletary at MD Anderson Cancer Center began a pilot project in 1999, and as of January 2001 had 13 patients undergo ablation prior to surgical resection.(26) RFA resulted in a complete tumor-cell kill in most patients. Both authors report that the procedure is extremely well tolerated, with few complications. The MD Anderson group have expanded this pilot to a multicenter study, and have plans to pilot a project to treat tumors less than 1.5cm in diameter with ablation alone followed by radiation therapy with a boost dose to the primary tumor site.(27)

Laser Interstitial Therapy

The use of laser energy for coagulation of breast tumors via an optic fiber was first described in 1983, (27) and has been utilized by several groups as a method of in situ ablation.(28, 29) A fiberoptic cable with a diffusing quartz tip is placed within the tumor. Either stereotactic guidance or MRI can be used for this. Light energy from the laser is passed through the cable and the resulting thermal energy can destroy the surrounding tissue over a radial region around the laser tip. The amount of laser energy needed to assure ablation is calculated based on the volume of the sphere surrounding the tumor, including a 0.5 cm cuff of normal breast tissue. Thermobprobes are placed percutaneously to monitor treatment and assure that the entire treatment area reaches 60°C.

Dowlatshahi et al have described the use of this technique to ablate breast tumors in 36 women with invasive or in situ tumors less than 2cm.(30, 31) The procedure was performed safely, with patients able to be discharged home with oral analgesics. All patients underwent surgical resection, and pathologic examination revealed complete necrosis in 24 of 36 patients (67%). The patients with residual tumor cells were felt to be due to technical failures, suboptimal target visualization and inadequate laser energy. They have also treated one cancer patient off protocol who refused surgical excision. She has not had a recurrence after two years.(27) Harms and colleagues have also reported their use of laser photocoagulation in breast cancer, with the use of MRI to determine the lesion extent and coordinate the therapy.(32) Thirty patients with breast cancer had 68 zones treated, with effective cell death in 60 zones (88%).

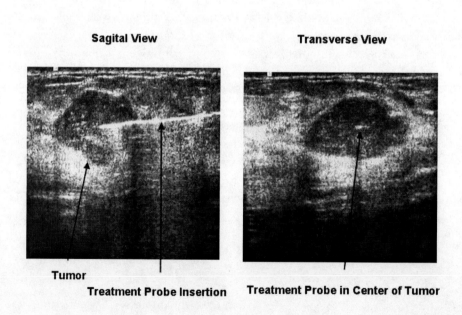

Sagital View   **Transverse View**

Tumor

Treatment Probe Insertion   **Treatment Probe in Center of Tumor**

Figure 13-4
Ultrasound images of breast tumor undergoing cryoablation. (Courtesy of Peter Littrup, M.D., Wayne State School of Medicine.

Cryosurgery

As opposed to radiofrequency ablation or laser interstitial therapy which use heat to destroy tumors, cryosurgery utilizes freezing temperatures. Cryosurgery for locally advanced breast carcinoma has been performed since the 1970's and has demonstrated therapeutic potential. Tanaka et al. treated 9 primary advanced breast cancer cases, and despite being inoperable, achieved long-term survival in 4 of the 9 patients.(33) Since then, the use of cryosurgery has been applied to the ablation of early-stage breast cancer.(34) Using ultrasound guidance, a cryoprobe, which is a metal probe with a freezing tip, can be placed into the center of the lesion.(Figure 4) An ice ball forms around the tumor which is monitored by ultrasound imaging. A 2-phase, or double, freeze-thaw cycle is employed to give maximal tumor cell death. Pfleiderer et al reported their results in 12 patients with primary breast tumors treated by cryosurgery.(35) Of 5 cases less than 1.5 cm, complete tumor-cell kill was obtained in each case. Incomplete necrosis was seen in 7 lesions larger than 2.3 cm.

Cryosurgery holds several potential benefits as a technique for the ablation of breast cancer. With cryoablation you can easily see the ice ball forming around the tumor, while with RFA or laser therapy it is less distinct at the periphery.(27) More importantly, it is possible that the mechanism of destruction in cryosurgery may allow for an immunologic response to the ablated tissue. After freezing there is local edema and initiation of the inflammatory cascade. This leads to macrophage invasion and resorption of the lesion. At this point, antigen presentation and the activation of specific T-cell and B-cell responses to tumor antigens may occur. As opposed to the coagulative necrosis seen with heat, freezing tissue does not denature the proteins and may induce their release from the membrane matrix.(36) This provides antigens for presentation and the generation of an immune response.

The suggestion that a cryoimmunologic benefit may exist came from clinical observations that patients being treated with cryosurgery showed regression of disease away from the primary tumor.(37-39) Suzuki described the regression of contralateral breast tumors and lymph node metastases in patients who underwent cryoablation of their inoperable primary breast cancer (39). The development of an anti-tumor immune response after cryosurgery for a variety of tumors has been demonstrated in both animal (40-42) and human trials.(39, 43-45)

High Intensity Focused Ultrasound

Radiofreqency, laser and cryoablation all require the placement of a probe within the mass of the tumor to achieve their results, hence they are minimally invasive. However, some technologies being investigated for the treatment of breast cancer are truly non-invasive. High-intensity focused ultrasound (FUS) utilizes intense, strongly focused ultrasound beams to heat tissues. With improved techniques for three-dimensional soft tissue imaging, FUS can obtain high spatial precision allowing for minimal destruction of normal tissue.(46, 47)

At the University of Arizona, FUS has been used for the treatment of a variety of malignancies, including 14 patients with locally advanced breast cancer or chest wall recurrences.(48) A planning simulation is performed prior to therapy to determine the most comfortable patient positioning and the optimal beam entry angles. During treatment, several diagnostic transducers are used to guide and monitor therapy while additional transducers deliver high intensity focussed ultrasound to heat the tissue. Intratumoral temperature probes are inserted percutaneously to make sure intratumoral temperatures reach at least 42.5oC for 30 minutes. Of the 14 breast patients treated, 5 (36%) achieved a complete response. Using MRI-guided FUS, Gianfelice et al. reported their experience treating patients with biopsy proven primary breast cancer who were not candidates for surgery.(49) While there was no histologic evaluation, 10 of 15 patients were rendered clinically tumor-free (evaluated by MRI and core biopsy) after one treatment with the remaining 5 patients to undergo repeat treatments. Additional trials utilizing focused ultrasound are underway for fibroadenomas (50) and early-stage cancers.(15)

Focused Microwave Thermotherapy

Another truly non-invasive method for the in situ ablation of breast cancer is Focused Microwave Thermotherapy (FMT). Based on technology originally developed to detect and destroy an enemy missile (known as the Strategic Defense Initiative or the Star Wars plan), it was discovered that this technology could be used to treat cancer cells.(51, 52) This technology takes advantage of the difference in water content between normal breast cells, which is 20 to 60% water, and cancer cells, which are typically around 80% water. Patients lie prone on a treatment table with two needle probes placed to sense and measure temperature changes during treatment. FMT can then be used to heat tumors to 46oC without burning the skin. Gardner et al. presented the results of a phase I trial where 10 women with advanced tumors underwent a single 20 to 40 minute microwave treatment.(53) A clinical response was seen in 60% of patients, and significant ischemic tumor necrosis was seen after mastectomy in 4 of 10 patients. One phase II trial is planned to combine FMT with preoperative chemotherapy while a second phase II trial will look at FMT alone to ablate early stage breast cancer.(14)

Role of Neoadjuvant Therapies

With the increased use of screening mammography, the average size of invasive tumors has decreased, increasing the proportion of patients who are candidates for breast conservation therapy.(54) However, a significant proportion of women still present with tumors too large relative to the size of their breast to be considered good candidates for lumpectomy. The use of neoadjuvant chemotherapy has been used with increased frequency to downstage these patients, and permit breast conservation therapy where it may have not otherwise been possible.

When the randomized clinical trials discussed above dispelled the Halstedian principle that the extent of surgical resection altered patient outcome, this not only shifted the emphasis of breast cancer treatment away from radical surgery towards breast conservation, but also established systemic therapy as an essential component. As the use of adjuvant chemotherapy became more widespread, the notion of delivering the chemotherapy prior to surgery arose. This approach had been utilized successfully for locally advanced cancers, allowing surgical resection for previously inoperable cancer.(55, 56) This same approach could potentially shrink large operable tumors, making breast conservation therapy available to women who would otherwise require mastectomy.(57) Several subsequent randomized trials demonstrated improved rates of breast conservation with the use of neoadjuvant chemotherapy.(58-60) The largest of these trials, NSABP B-18, randomized 1523 women to receive four cycles of AC either before or after surgery.(61) All women 50 years of age or older received 5 years of tamoxifen after completion of chemotherapy. There were no significant differences in disease free survival, distant disease free survival or overall survival between the two groups. Women who received preoperative chemotherapy were more likely to undergo a lumpectomy than were women who received postoperative chemotherapy (67% versus 60%, p= 0.002) and this was more dramatic in women with larger tumors.

While neoadjuvant chemotherapy is not superior to standard adjuvant chemotherapy in the B-18 trial, because it is not worse, there are potential advantages that warrant its use. Most obviously, the use of neoadjuvant chemotherapy as a method to make breast conservation therapy available to women whom might otherwise require mastectomy. In the future, neoadjuvant chemotherapy may be used to down stage women requiring lumpectomy, so that they are candidates for in situ ablation. In addition to the cosmetic benefits, as our understanding of the biology of breast cancer grows, and the technology for screening, diagnosis and treatment improves, the role of neoadjuvant therapies in the future will become standard approaches.

The genomic expression of individual breast tumors will identify unique targets which will help guide the choice of systemic therapies that can be employed. For example, breast cancers will be found to have specific receptors that are present of their cell surface that can serve as targets for the immune system. An example of such a receptor is Her2/neu which has been found to be a useful prognostic factor as well as predictor for response to alkylating agents. Furthermore, an antibody to this receptor, HerceptinR, has been found to be therapeutic when administered in conjunction with chemotherapeutic agents. Identification of other surface tumor-associated antigens will lead to the development of other antibodies that can be conjugated with tumoricidal reagents for therapy. These antigens can also be employed in vaccine strategies for the treatment of bulk disease (ie., in the neoadjuvant setting) or in the micrometastatic setting (post-ablative adjuvant therapy).

Another role genomic profiling will be useful in will be to identify intracellular targets for therapy. Identification of unique cell signaling pathways in cancers will lead to new agents that can block those pathways. One excellent example is the identification of STI-571 (GleevacR) as an active agent in chronic myelogenous leukemia and gastrointestinal stromal tumors. In these tumor types, the presence of c-kit tyrosinase as a signaling pathway lead to the discovery that a small molecule can block it and result in tumor cell death.(62) It is predicted that other examples of this therapeutic approach will be identified for a variety of malignancies, including breast cancer.

Future of Reconstructive Surgery

Despite the advances in local control of breast cancers that will be seen in the future, many women will still require mastectomy. Due to multi-focal disease or previous history of local radiotherapy, many breast cancer patients will not be candidates for breast conservation. Even in the absence of these contraindications, some women still favor mastectomy for treatment of their disease. Despite predictions in recent years of mastectomy's demise as a therapeutic option, it remains a common choice for patients and providers. While mastectomy has persisted as a standard treatment for breast cancer, breast reconstruction following mastectomy has seen considerable growth over the last twenty years, due in part to technical innovations and to growing public awareness of reconstructive options. The increasing popularity of breast reconstruction can also be attributed to recent studies demonstrating the psychosocial and quality of life benefits of these procedures.(63)

Current practice in breast reconstruction is largely based on three major innovations in plastic surgery over the past two decades: tissue expansion, musculocutaneous flaps, and microsurgical tissue transfers. Future progress in breast reconstruction appears most likely in the area of autogenous (or natural) tissue techniques, rather than in prosthetic implants. This trend towards autogenous tissue reconstructions and away from implants can be attributed to recent public and governmental concerns over the safety of prosthetic implants. Natural tissue approaches also offer opportunities for greater flexibility and creativity in meeting the technical demands of breast reconstruction. Further innovations may focus on development of flaps which harvest the skin and adipose tissue needed for creation of a new breast without muscle sacrifice and the associated potential for functional deficits. Unlike the current transverse rectus abdominis musculocutaneous (TRAM) flap, which may leave its abdominal donor site with structural or functional complications, newer flaps for breast reconstruction may be harvested with little or no adverse effect. Recently, several of these new-generation flaps have been described: Allen and colleagues have proposed a deep inferior epigastric artery (DIEP) flap which, like the conventional TRAM technique, harvests the lower abdominal skin and fat for breast reconstruction but avoids sacrificing any muscle tissue.(64) Similarly, an inferior gluteal perforator flap has been described which uses skin and fat from the lower buttock area as donor tissues for mastectomy reconstruction. Undoubtedly, additional new sources and designs for flaps will be devised for breast reconstruction in coming years.

In the future, the rapidly evolving field of tissue engineering is likely to impact many areas of plastic surgery, including breast reconstruction. Originally, research in tissue engineering focused on culturing cells in vitro on two dimensional substrates and, subsequently, on three dimensional lattices for eventual implantation.(65) More recently, investigators have been studying the use of porous absorbable matrices seeded with cells and growth factors, which regulate tissue growth. These devices are implanted in vivo as frameworks for tissue generation. Use of this technology could reproduce an infinite variety of breast shapes and sizes, without donor site complications. However, before these innovations become clinically practical, a number of challenges must be overcome. Not least among these issues is the identification of an optimal matrix to promote and direct cell growth. The ideal framework for a tissue-engineered breast must be sufficiently rigid to mold cell growth into a natural shape, but also soft enough to simulate a natural breast. Maintenance of the breast contour over time also remains an obstacle.

The future of breast reconstruction will be guided by technical innovations but will also be impacted by numerous health policy and funding challenges. With passage of the Women's Cancer and Health Rights Act of 1997, Federal law requires inclusion of breast reconstruction services as covered benefits for all health care plans in the United States. Despite this mandate, a recent analysis of the Surveillance, Epidemiology, and End Results (SEER) database for 11 major regions in the U.S. indicated that most mastectomy patients still are not receiving reconstruction. In 1998, only 15% of the 10,406 database patients treated with mastectomy underwent reconstruction within four months of the mastectomy. A four-fold variation in rates of reconstruction was seen between the region with the highest rate (Atlanta) and the area with the lowest utilization (Hawaii). Significant variation in rates also was noted among ethnic groups: Compared with Caucasian women, African-Americans were less than half as likely to receive reconstruction, while Asian-Americans were less than one third as likely to be reconstructed.(66)

Etiologies for the low utilization of reconstruction observed among mastectomy patients, as well as for the wide variations in rates of this procedure, are uncertain. With reimbursement rates for reconstruction on the decline, financial barriers likely play important roles in these findings. In many regions, third party payers cover only a fraction of the total cost of reconstruction, with patients being required to foot the remainder of the bill. Thus, women who are unable to contribute substantially to the costs of care are often frustrated in their attempts to obtain reconstruction. Additional reforms on a national level may be required to ensure not only that health care plans offer reconstruction as a covered benefit, but also that payers provide sufficient funding to cover the actual costs of these procedures.

Access to reconstruction following mastectomy also may be hampered by a lack of patient awareness that such options exist. New educational interventions by health care organizations may be required to provide patients with up-to-date, understandable information about reconstructive choices. Initiatives are currently underway to develop patient education programs through the use of Internet, CD-ROM, and other technologies. Finally, new research and policy initiatives will be required to address ethnic disparities in utilization of breast reconstruction following mastectomy. Identifying and overcoming cultural barriers to care could help ensure that breast reconstruction and its quality of life benefits are available to underserved populations. The coming decades will likely see numerous technical advances in mastectomy reconstruction. An additional goal should be providing access to these services for any patient who needs them.

Role of Chemoprevention and Vaccines in the Future

Within this past decade, there have been significant advances in the area of chemoprevention of breast cancer. There is compelling evidence that the total life time exposure of an individual to estrogen is associated with the development of breast cancer. In trials of tamoxifen as adjuvant therapy, it was observed that there was a significant reduction of women developing second primary cancers in the contralateral breast. Tamoxifen is one of several drugs that are classified as selective estrogen receptor modulators (SERMs). SERMs are pharacologic agents which produce estrogenic and/or anti-estrogenic effects at different sites in a woman's body. Based upon these observations, the National Surgical Adjuvant Breast and Bowel Project (NSABP) conducted a randomized clinical trial (P-1) to assess the chemoprevention efficacy of tamoxifen in women without breast cancer.(67) This trial was open to women 60 years of age or older, or women with known lobular carcinoma in situ, or women 35-59 years of age with a 5-year predicted risk for breast cancer of at least 1.66%. Eligible subjects were randomized to receive tamoxifen (20mg/day) versus placebo for 5 years. A total of 13,388 women were entered. Tamoxifen reduced the risk of invasive breast cancer by 49% (p<0.00001) with a cumulative incidence through 69 months of follow-up of 43.4 versus 22.0 per 1000 women in the placebo and tamoxifen groups, respectively. Tamoxifen reduced the occurrence of estrogen receptor-positive tumors by 69%, but no difference in the occurrence of estrogen receptor-negative tumors was seen. The rate of endometrial cancer and rates of stroke and venous thrombosis was increased in the group that received tamoxifen. Despite these side-effects, it was concluded that the use of tamoxifen as a preventive agent was appropriate in many women at increased risk for the disease.

Raloxifene is a SERM that has been shown to increase bone density in postmenopausal women and is currently indicated for the prevention and treatment of osteoporosis in this population.(68) A meta-analysis of data combined from several randomized placebo-controlled trials of raloxifene was completed.(69) The trials were not conducted to look at breast cancer risk reduction as a primary end-point. Nevertheless, in a total of 10,533 postmenopausal women with no personal history of breast cancer, the risk reduction for all breast cancers was 0.46 with raloxifene. In the placebo group, there were 3.7 cases of breast cancer per thousand women compared with 1.7 cases per thousand women in the raloxifene-treated group. Since raloxifene may be associated with fewer side-effects, the NSABP is currently conducting a trial to evaluate raloxifene vs. tamoxifen as a chemopreventive regimen in up to 22,000 women P-2 study.

The raloxifene and tamoxifen trials have already demonstrated the ability to reduce the risk of breast cancer by the administration of targeted agents (ie. SERMs) in women. This approach has reduced the risk of estrogen-receptor positive breast cancers but not estrogen-receptor negative cancers. A complementary approach to reduce the risk of the latter may be the use of vaccines in the foreseeable future. Based upon the findings from genomic and proteomic research, it is anticipated that many new targets associated with the development of breast cancer will be identified. This should allow the development of vaccines which consist of multiple breast cancer associated antigens that can be administered to block the induction of breast cancer. Recently, the use of a multi-epitope vaccine has been found to significantly improve disease-free survival in melanoma patients in the adjuvant setting.(70) This latter study is proof of principle that a vaccine approach in humans is effective in preventing the growth of micrometastatic disease and sets the stage for vaccines in other tumor types.

There are a variety of tumor vaccines that are being tested in clinical settings. A list of the types of vaccines under investigation are summarized in Table 1. One of the earliest vaccines to be studied were autologous tumor cell vaccines. These have the advantages of containing all the relevant tumor antigens to which the individual patient can be immunized against. However, a major drawback is the availability of such tumor cells in every patient. The presence of shared tumor antigens expressed on tumors of the same histology (ie, melanoma) paved the way for the use of allogeneic tumor cells as vaccine sources. Allogeneic cell lines can be immortalized and grown in large batch quantities for use in the general population. One drawback of using mixtures of allogeneic cell lines is the possibility that the vaccine won't contain relevant tumor rejection antigens that would cover all patients. Purified antigens are also being explored in clinical studies. These represent known tumor-associated antigens for specific tumor histologies that are usually combined with an immune adjuvant to increase their immunogenicity. The advantage of purified antigens relates to their availability as a synthesized product that can readily be quality-controlled, and the ability to monitor immune responses to specific antigens. In the future, each newly diagnosed breast cancer will be evaluated by proteomic techniques to determine what tumor-associated antigens are expressed by the tumor. Once the profile of antigens are identified, a clinician will be able to retrieve several of these synthesized antigens off the shelf for vaccine use. Recently, the use of dendritic cells as a cellular vaccine has been drawing a lot of interest. Dendritic cells (DC) are capable of processing and presenting to naive T cells tumor antigen in a variety of forms. Clinical trials are underway to assess the efficacy of these vaccines in the advanced disease setting.(71-73) Based upon their efficiency in eliciting immune responses, it is predicted that DC will be an important component of vaccine therapy in the future and will be used as vehicles for antigens to be presented to the patient. Lastly, several investigations are underway to examine the utility of genetically modified cell-based vaccines. By inserting immunostimulatory genes into cell-based vaccines (ie., autologous tumor, allogeneic tumor or DC) one will enhance their effectiveness in eliciting an immune response in the host. The current regulatory climate regarding these types of vaccines is too restrictive to consider this a practical approach at this time.

Summary

The revolution of discovery since the mapping of the human genome is just beginning. The use of genomics and proteomics will establish new systems to classify and stage cancers. This will eliminate the need for axillary staging. With molecular techniques, tailored treatment approaches based upon the individual tumors sampled from patients will become standard. Neoadjuvant therapy to enhance the ability to perform breast-sparing treatment will be employed more often in the immediate future. The focus of surgical therapy will be local control of the primary tumor. More use of incision-less therapies will be used to control the primary, and the surgeon will need to learn the techniques of the interventional radiologist to keep pace with the field. Tissue engineering advances will provide alternative reconstruction options for women who do require mastectomy. Based upon current trends of prevention, it is predicted that breast cancer will become a rare disease.

REFERENCES

1. Halsted WS. The results of operations for the cure of cancer of the breast performed at the Johns Hopkins Hospital from June 1889, to January, 1894. Annals of Surgery 1894; 20: 497-555.

2. Veronesi U, Saccozzi R, Del Vecchio M, et al. Comparing radical mastectomy with quadrantectomy, axillary dissection, and radiotherapy in patients with small cancers of the breast. The New England Journal of Medicine 1981; 305(1): 6-11.

3. Fisher B, Bauer M, Margolese R, et al. Five-year results of a randomized clinical trial comparing total mastectomy and segmental mastectomy with or without radiation in the treatment of breast cancer. The New England Journal of Medicine 1985; 312(11): 665-681.

4. Fisher B, Redmond C, Poisson R, et al. Eight-year results of randomized clinical trial comparing total mastectomy and lumpectomy with or without irradiation in the treatment of breast cancer. The New England Journal of Medicine 1989; 320(13): 822-828.

5. Collins F, Guyer MS, Peterson J, et al. Initial sequencing and analysis of the human genome. Nature 2001; 409: 860-921.

6. Venter CJ, Adams MD, Myers EW, et al. The sequence of the human genome. Science 2001; 291: 1304-1351.

7. Collins FS McKusick V, A. Implications of the human genome project for medical science. The Journal of the American Medical Association 2001; 285(5): 540-544.

8. Futreal AP, Kasprzyk A, Birney E, et al. Cancer and genomics. Nature 2001; 409: 850-852.

9. Sørlie T, Perou CM, Tibshirani R, et al. Gene Expression patterns of breast carcinomas distinguish tumor subclasses with clinical implications. Proceedings of the National Academy of Sciences 2001; 98(19): 10869-10874.

10. van't Veer L, Dai H, van de Vijver M, et al. Gene expression profiling predicts clinical outcome of breast cancer. Nature 2002; 415: 530-536.

11. Hedenfalk I, Duggan D, Chen Y, et al. Gene-expression profiles in hereditary breast cancer. The New England Journal of Medicine 2001; 344(8): 539-548.

12. Unger MA, Rishi M, Clemmer VB, et al. Characterization of adjacent breast tumors using oligonucleotide microarrays. Breast Cancer Research 2001; 3: 336-341.

13. Bichsel VE, Liotta LA Petricoin EFI. Cancer Proteomics: From biomarker discovery to signal pathway profiling. The Cancer Journal 2001; 7(1): 69-78.

14. Sabel MS Edge SB. In-Situ ablation of breast cancer. Breast Disease 2001; 12(1): 131-140.

15. Singletary SE. Minimally invasive techniques in breast cancer treatment. Seminars in Surg Onc 2001; 20: 246-250.

16. Curley SA. Radiofrequency ablation of malignant liver tumors. Oncologist 2001; 6(1): 14-23.

17. McGhana JP Dodd GD, III. Radiofrequency ablation of the liver: current status. AJR 2001; 176(1): 3-16.

18. Mirza AN, Fornage BD, Sneige N, et al. Radiofrequency ablation of solid tumors. Cancer Journal 2001; 7(2): 95-102.

19. Zlotta AR, Djavan B, Matos, et al. Percutaneous transperineal radiofrequency ablatoin of prostate tumor: safety, feasibility and pathological effects on human prostate cancer. British Journal of Urology 1998; 81: 265.

20. Rosenthal DI, Horniecek FJ, Wolfe MW, et al. Percutaneous radiofrequency coagulation of osteoid osteoma compared with operative treatment. J Bone Joint Surg Am 1998; 80: 815-821.

21. Zlotta AR, Wildschutz T, Raviv G, et al. Radiofrequency interstitial tumor ablation (RITA) is a possible new modality for treatment of renal cancer; ex vivo and in vivo experience. J Endourol 1997; 11: 251-258.

22. Goldberg SN, Kruskal JB, Oliver BS, et al. Percutaneous tumor ablation: increased coagulation by combining radio-frequency ablation and ethanol instillation in rat breast tumor model. Radiology 2000; 217(3): 827-831.

23. McGahan JP, Griffey SM, Schneider PD, et al. Radiofrequency electrocautery ablation of mammary tissue in swine. Radiology 2000; 217(2): 471-476.

24. Jeffrey SS, Birdwell RL, Ideda DM, et al. Radiofrequency ablation of breast cancer: First report of an emerging technology. Arch Surg 1999; 134: 1064-1068.

25. Izzo F, Thomas R, Delrio P, et al. Radiofrequency ablation in patients with primary breast carcinoma: a pilot study in 26 patients. Cancer 2001; 92(8): 2036-44.

26. Singletary SE. Minimally invasive techniques in breast cancer treatment. Seminars in Surgical Oncology 2001; 20: 246-250.

27. Simmons RM, Dowlatshahi K, Singletary SE, et al. Symposium: Image-guided ablation of breast tumors. Contemporary Surgery 2002; 58(2): 61-71.

28. Harries SA, Amin Z, Smith ME, et al. Interstitial laser photocoagulation as a treatment for breast cancer. Br. J. Surg 1998; 81: 1617-1619.

29. Robinson DS, Parel JM, Denham DB, et al. Stereotactic uses beyond core biopsy: model development for minimally invasive treatment of breast cancer through interstitial laser hyperthermia. Am Surg 1996; 62: 117-118.

30. Dowlatshahi K, Fan M, Gould VE, et al. Stereotactically guided laser therapy of occult breast tumors; Work in progress report. Arch Surg 2000; 135: 1345-1352.

31. Dowlatshahi K, Fan M, Shekarloo M, et al. Stereotaxic interstitial laser therapy of early-stage breast cancer. Breast J 1996; 2: 304-311.

32. Harms SE, Klimberg VS, Henry-Tilllman R, et al. MRI directed laser therapy for benign and malignant breast neoplasms: Clinical follow-up and histologic correlation. (Absract). Radiological Society of North American 2000 Annual Meeting 2000; .

33. Tanaka S. Cryosurgical treatment of advanced breast cancer. Skin Cancer 1995; 10: 9-18.

34. Staren ED, Sabel MS, Gianakakis LM, et al. Cryosurgery of breast cancer. Arch Surg 1997; 132: 28-34.

35. Pfleiderer SO, Freeesmeyer MG, Fleck M, et al. Ultrasound-guided cryosurgery of breast cancer: first results (Absract). Radiological Society of North America Meeting 2000; .

36. Roy A, Sobhendranath G, Lahiri S, et al. Some aspects of the causes of enhanced immune responses of in vitro frozen ascites fibrosarcoma tumor cells in mice. Cryobiology 1995; 32: 306-313.

37. Gage AA. Cryosurgery for oral and pharyngeal carcinoma. Am J. Surg 1969; 118: 669-672.

38. Soanes WA, Ablin RJ Gonder MJ. Remission of metastatic lesions following cryosurgery in prostatic cancer. J Urol 1970; 104: 154-159.

39. Suzuki Y. Cryosurgical treatment of advanced breast cancer and cyroimmunological responses. Skin Cancer 1995; 10: 19-26.

40. Blackwood CE Cooper IS. Response of experimental tumor systems to cryosurgery. Cryobiology 1972; 9: 508-515.

41. Jacob G, Li AKC Hobbs KEF. A comparison of cryodestruction with excision or infarction of implanted tumor in rat liver. Cryobiology 1984; 21: 148-156.

42. Misao A, Sakata K, Saji S, et al. Late appearance of resistance to tumor rechallenge following cryosurgery. Cryobiology 1981; : 386-389.

43. Fazio M, Airoldi M, Gandolfo S, et al. Humoral and cellular immune response to cryosurgery of benign and malignant lesions of the oral cavity. Bollettino-Society Italiana Biologia Sperimentale 1982; 58(7): 412-418.

44. Wang ZS. Cryosurgery in rectal carcinoma-report of 41 cases. Chinese Journal of Oncology 1989; 11(3): 226-227.

45. Kogel H, Grunmann R, Fohlmeister I, et al. Cryotherapy of rectal cancer. Immunologic results. Zentralblatt fur Chirurgie 1985; 110((2-3)): 147-154.

46. Hill CR Haar GR. High intensity focused ultrasound-potential for cancer treatment. Br J Radiol 1995; 68: 1296-1303.

47. Cline HE, Hynyen KH Roemer RB. Focused US system for MR imaging-guided tumor ablation. Radiology 1995; 194(3): 731-737.

48. Harari PM, Hynynen KH, Roemer RB, et al. Development of scanned focussed ultrasound hyperthermia: Clinical response evaluation. Int. J Radio Oncol Biol Phys 1991; 21: 831-840.

49. Gianfelice DC, Hail M Lepanto L. Initial treatment protocol for breast neoplasms with MR-guided focused ultrasound ablation (MR-FUS) apparatus: Works in Progress (Abstract). in Radiological Society of North America 85th Annual Meeting. 1999. Chicago, IL.

50. Hynyen K, Pomeroy O Smith DN. MR Imaging-guided focused ultrasound surgery of fibroadenomas in the breast: A feasibility study. Radiology 2001; 219(1): 176-185.

51. Fenn AJ, Sathiaseelan V, King GA, et al. Improved localization of energy depostion in adaptive phased-array hyperthermia treatment of cancer. Linconl Laboratory Journal 1996; 9(2): 187-196.

52. Fenn AJ, Wolf GL Fogle RM. An adaptive microwave phased array for targeted heating of deep tumors in intact breast: animal study results. Int J Hyperthermia 1999; 15(1): 45-61.

53. Gardner RA, Vargas HI, Block CL, et al. Focused microwave phased array (FMPA) thermotherapy for primary breast cancer (Abstract). SSO 54th Annual Cancer Symposium Abstract Book 2001; : 40.

54. Hunt KK Ross MI, Changing trends in the diagnosis and treatment of early breast cancer. Pollock R, ed. Surgical Oncology. 1997, Boston: Kluwer Academic Publishers. 171-201.

55. Schick P, Goodstein J, Moor J, et al. Preoperative chemotherapy followed by mastectomy for locally advanced breast cancer. J Surg Oncol 1983; 22: 278-282.

56. Sorace RA, Bagley CS, Lichter AS, et al. The management of nonmetastatic locally advanced breast cancer using primary induction chemotherapy with hormonal synchronization followed by radiation therapy with or without debulking surgery. World J Surg 1985; 9: 775-785.

57. Bonadonna G, Veronesi U, Brambilla C, et al. Primary chemotherapy to avoid mastectomy in tumors with diameters of three centimeters or more. J Natl Cancer Inst 1990; 82: 1539-1545.

58. Mauriac L, Durand M, Avril A, et al. Effects on primary chemotherapy in conservative treatment of breast cancer patients with operable tumors larger than 3 cm. Ann Oncol 1991; 2: 347-354.

59. Scholl SM, Fourquet A, Asselain B, et al. Neoadjuvant versus adjuvant chemotherapy in premenopausal patients with tumors considered too large for breast conserving surgery. Preliminary results of a randomized trial. Eur J Cancer 1994; 30: 645-652.

60. Powles TJ, Hickish TF, Makris A, et al. Randomized trial of chemoendocrine therapy started before or after surgery for treatment of primary breast cancer. J Clin Oncol 1995; 13: 547-552.

61. Fisher B, Brown A, Mamounas E, et al. Effect of preoperative chemotherapy of local-regional disease in women with operable breast cancer. Findings from national Surgical Adjuvant Breast and Bowel Project B18. J Clinical Oncol 1997; 15: 2483-2493.

62. Druker B Lydon NB. Lessons learned from the development of an Ab1 tryosine kinase inhibitor for chronic myelogenous leukemia. The Journal of Clinical Investigation 2000; 105(1): 3-7.

63. Wilkins EG, Cederna PS, Lowery JC, et al. Prospective analysis of psychosocial outcomes in breast reconstruction: One year postoperative results of the Michigan breast reconstruction outcome study. Plastic and Reconstructive Surgery 2000; 106: 1014.

64. Allen RJ Treece P. Deep inferior epigastric perforator flap for breast reconstruction. Annals of Plastic Surgery 1994; 32: 32-38.

65. Langer R Vacanti JP. Tissue Engineering. Science 1993; 260: 920-926.

66. Alderman AA, ., McMahon L Wilkins EG. Utilization of immediate reconstruction in the U.S. and the impact of sociodemographic factors. Plastic and Reconstructive Surgery .

67. Fisher B, Costantino JP, Wickerham LD, et al. Tamoxifen for prevention of breast cancer: Report of the National Surgical Adjuvant Breast and Bowel Project P1 Study. Journal of the National Cancer Institute 1998; 90(18): 1371-1388.

68. Cummings SR, Eckert S, Krueger K, et al. The effect of raloxifene on risk of breast cancer in postmenopausal women: Results from the MORE randomized trial. JAMA 1999; 281(23): 2189-2197.

69. Pritchard KI. Selective estrogen receptor modulators in the prevention and treatment of breast cancer. Clinical Oncology 2001; 3(4): 1-15.

70. Sosman JA, Unger JM, Liu P-Y, et al. Adjuvant immunotherapy of resected, intermediate-thickness, node-negative melanoma with an allogeneic tumor vaccine: Impact of HLA class I antigen expression on outcome. Journal of Clinical Oncology 2002; 20: 2067-2075.

71. Nestle FO, Alijagic S, Gilliet M, et al. Vaccination of melanoma patients with peptide- or tumor lysate-pulsed dendritic cells. Nature Med. 1998; 4(3): 328-332.

72. Chang AE, Redman B, G., Whitfield JR, et al. A phase I trial of tumor lysate-pulsed dendritic cells in the treatment of advanced cancer. Clinical Cancer Research 2002; 8: 1021-1032..

73. Panelli MC, Wunderlich J, Jeffries J, et al. Phase 1 study in patients with metastatic melanoma of immunization with dendritic cells presenting epitopes derived from the melanoma-associated antigens MART-1 and gp 100. Journal of Immunotherapy 2000; 23(4): 487-498.

Table 1. Tumor Vaccine Classification

Type	Advantages	Disadvantages
1. Autologous tumor cells	Will express all potential tumor rejection antigens for individual patient.	Not available in all patients
2. Allogeneic tumor cells	Since these represent cell lines, availability in not an issue.	May not contain the important rejection antigens for individual patient.
3. Purified antigens (ie. peptides, glycoproteins, carbohydrates)	Can be synthetically manufactured. Easy to use as off-the-shelf reagent.	May not represent the important tumor rejection antigens for individual patient.
4. Dendritic cells	Can process and present cell-based antigens (ie., tumor cells), peptides or DNA-encoded antigens.	Optimal maturation state of DC and route of administration not yet defined.
5. Gene-modified cell-based vaccines	Immunostimulatory genes can enhance the effectiveness of a particular cell-based vaccine.	Identification of appropriate immunostimulatory genes and toxicity profiles need to be established. Regulatory concerns can be very restrictive

CHAPTER 14

TRANSPLANT SURGERY

JEFFREY D. PUNCH, M.D.

Organ transplantation is a relatively new discipline. In the span of the last quarter of a century, transplantation has been transformed from an experimental procedure that rarely succeeded in prolonging the patient's life, to the standard of care for end stage organ failure due to chronic renal, hepatic, cardiac, and pulmonary diseases. The current success of organ transplantation has been primarily the result of advances in immunosuppression that now allow acceptance of transplanted organs in the majority of cases. Graft rejection, once the expected consequence of transplanting foreign grafts into immuno-competent hosts, is now the exception. An enhanced capability to reverse established rejection means that graft loss due to acute rejection is now rare. The toxic, nonspecific, drugs that were used in the 1960's and 1970's have been largely replaced with agents that are engineered to specifically alter immunologic responses associated with allograft rejection, while leaving the arms of the immune system that protect the recipient from infectious diseases intact. Together with improvements in organ preservation techniques, improved understanding of infectious diseases associated with chronic immunosuppression, and technical advances, modern immunosuppression resulted in a major growth in the number of organs transplanted in the 1990's (Figure 1).

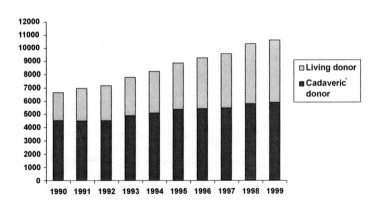

Figure 14-1
All solid organ transplants per year in the U.S.

169

Unfortunately, the spectacular clinical success of organ transplantation has been marred by the fact that the supply of transplantable organs has not been able to keep pace with demand. As success rates rose and methods improved, indications expanded and the number of patients that were candidates for life saving transplants grew. The result has been a national shortage of organs, and consequently a waiting list mortality rate that continues to rise. Despite significant legislative efforts to promote organ donation, the number of the number of patients waiting for organs has increased radically.(Figure 2) In order to meet the unmet need for organs, new techniques and strategies continue to be developed. This chapter will discuss several of these new procedures, with particular emphasis on how they will impact the design of the 21st century operating room.

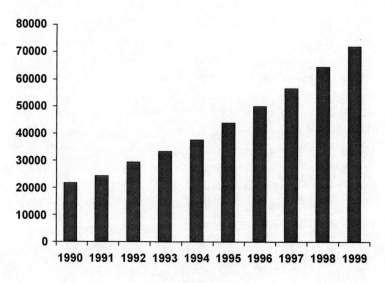

Figure 14-2
Number of patients waiting for solid organ transplants in the U.S.

Laparoscopic Kidney Donation

In 1996 the group at Johns Hopkins reported three cases of laparoscopic living donor nephrectomy.(1) As with laparoscopic cholecystectomy, the procedure was heralded as a method of reducing pain associated with the procedure, and hence the recovery time from the operation. Indeed, early reports indicated significantly less morbidity associated with the laparoscopic procedure when compared to standard living donor nephrectomy through a flank incision.(2) It was thus argued that this procedure would increase the pool of live kidney donors since decreased morbidity would allow the donor to return to usual activities, including employment, sooner. However, similar to laparoscopic cholecystectomy a decade earlier, few rigorous studies to determine the relative benefit of the procedure compared to the standard of care were undertaken. The procedure rapidly gained popularity, particularly in competitive markets where word spread rapidly of the new procedure that allowed one to donate a kidney with reduced pain and suffering.

Some surgeons remained skeptical that the benefit of laparoscopic nephrectomy was as great as claimed. Theoretical arguments have been raised that the outcome following laparoscopic nephrectomy may not be as good due to the decreased renal blood flow that is associated with pneumoperitoneum. In addition, the transperitoneal nature of standard laparoscopy means that the donor will be at risk for later bowel obstruction, a complication that does not occur following the open nephrectomy using an extra-peritoneal flank approach.(3) Intuitively, the advantage of a laparoscopic donor nephrectomy over a standard nephrectomy would seem to be limited by the requirement for an incision large enough to remove a kidney intact.

When studied in a randomized and controlled manner with careful assessment of pain and disability, the laparoscopic procedure did appear to provide a tangible benefit compared to open nephrectomy.(4) Also comforting are several large series that report excellent clinical results, with low rates of delayed graft function.(5, 6). Until a comprehensive donor registry is available with long term follow-up, it will be impossible to judge the relative safety of the procedure, especially as it is practiced around the country by surgeons at programs with both low and high volumes. The procedure continues to gain popularity, and has become the primary method of performing living donor nephrectomy at many kidney transplant centers. Whether it has actually increased the number of willing living donors is difficult to know.

Laparoscopic living donor nephrectomy is a more technically challenging procedure than open nephrectomy. It also takes significantly longer to perform. Prior to the institution of laparoscopic nephrectomy it was standard procedure to begin the recipient operation 30 to 45 minutes after the donor operation was begun. In this way the donor kidney would be out of the donor and perfused at about the same time that the recipient team would be ready for the kidney. A much longer delay is necessary before the recipient is anesthetized when the donor operation is to be done laparoscopically. In a randomized trial, operative time was 65% longer in the laparoscopy group (4). In order to efficiently utilize operating time it is standard procedure now to schedule a dialysis access operation in the operating room where the recipient's operation will occur. There is ample time available before the recipient operation needs to begin for a procedure that lasts 1 to 2 hours.

Despite the increased operative time, there was 47% less analgesic use, 35% shorter hospital stay, 33% more rapid return to non-strenuous activity, and 73%

less pain six weeks post-operatively in the laparoscopic group compared to the open surgical group of the randomized trial. While overall mean hospital cost was 24% greater in the laparoscopy group, global cost, which included estimated loss of occupational income during the recovery period, was only 2% greater in the laparoscopy group. Residual effects more than six months following the operation were reported by 11% of the laparoscopic patients and 90% of the open surgical patients. Thus, despite the increased operating room cost associated with laparoscopic nephrectomy due to the non-reusable instruments and due to the increased operative time required, it was found that the decreased length of stay return to work compensated for operating room cost (7). Patients frequently seek out centers that offer laparoscopic living kidney donation due to the perceived benefits. This perception may be exaggerated, but when a healthy donor is facing a painful procedure that they do not need, it is not surprising that they elect to find the method that will result in the least personal suffering.

Living Related Hepatic Transplantation- Left Lateral Segment Grafts

The increased demand for organs and the relatively flat donation rate have resulted in progressively longer waiting times for cadaveric organs.(Figure 3) This delay, in turn, has resulted in progressively rising mortality rates for patients waiting.(Figure 4) The need for organs has been the predominant factor resulting in the development of living donation techniques. In the case of kidney transplantation, the first successful transplants were from living donors. In the case of liver transplantation, the first successful living donor transplant was reported in 1989.(8) This transplant involved the removal of the left lateral segment of a healthy adult for transplantation to a child. Prior to the broad adoption of this technique in the United States, the procedure was first discussed in theoretical terms.(9) It was the general conclusion of the transplant community that the removal of a left lateral segment graft could be done safely, and that informed consent was possible, despite the obvious conflict of interest on the part of the donor- who is often the parent of the recipient. Led by the excellent results reported by the University of Chicago, the technique spread throughout the world.(10)

It rapidly became evident that the technique of transplanting the left lateral segment of an adult donor was limited because the segment only provided sufficient hepatic mass for pediatric recipients. This technique had a substantial impact on the ability of children to receive a liver transplant before either dying, or becoming extremely ill, although the technique does not appear superior to that obtained with an appropriately sized match graft.(11) In recent years, living related donation for pediatric recipients has fallen in some areas due to the availability of split liver grafts from cadaver donors.(12) This technique has become the preferred method of providing grafts for small children at some centers, and will be discussed in a later section.

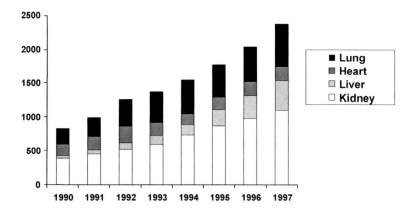

Figure 14-3
Median waiting time for solid organ transplants in the U.S.

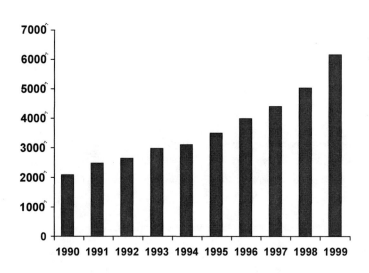

Figure 14-4
Deaths while waiting for solid organ transplants in the U.S.

Despite the limited applicability of left lateral segment living donor transplantation, it is clear that the technique is here to stay, and will continue to impact operating room needs. The living donor operation averages 4.5 hours. Since most cadaveric organs are procured at outside hospitals, living donor transplantation does tend to increase overall operating room utilization at the transplant center. This factor is off-set by the fact that the operations are done electively in the majority of cases, which makes the feat logistically easier to some degree.

Living Related Hepatic Transplantation- Right Lobe Grafts

The success rate achieved with living donor liver transplantation in children us-ing left lateral segment grafts soon led to the desire to procure an organ large enough for an adult recipient from a living donor. Unlike the situation when living donor liver transplantation using left lateral segments was begun, the transition to using right lobe grafts was not debated before it was initiated. This probably occurred for three reasons. First, the need for livers had become progressively more dire. Second, the left lateral segment living donor procedure had been broadly accepted by the medical community and the general public as both a medically effective, and an ethi-cally justifiable practice. Finally, the procedure of right lobe living donor donation was initially popularized in Japan, where cadaveric donation is not practiced to any significant degree.(13) Due in part to the fact that living donation was the only op-tion in this part of the world, cases series soon began to appear from Japan.(14) Very quickly the technique spread to the United States and Europe.

Recently, concerns have been raised regarding the ethics of right lobe donation. While the core principle of human autonomy appears to primarily underlie the ap-propriateness of allowing a healthy person to undergo an operation with an approxi-mate morality of one percent, issues have been raised regarding whether all centers that are performing the procedure are adequately qualified, and whether all potential donors are fully appraised of the risks they face. Calls for national oversight are be-ing made. In addition, it is very clear that a donor registry to accurately track donor complications will be necessary in order to provide prospective donors with mean-ingful estimates of the risks that donation entails. Nevertheless, it appears likely that the practice will continue, and almost certainly will become more common in the future.

The growing practice of living donor liver transplantation will impact the op-erating suite in several ways, some positive and some negative. First, the fact that living donor transplants can be scheduled during daylight hours makes the procedure somewhat easier from an operating room staffing point of view. However, the fact that the donor requires their own operative suite and team essentially doubles the overall operating room utilization time. Right lobe donation typically requires six or more hours to complete. An additional factor that must be considered is that as living donor transplants become more commonplace it will be necessary for liver transplant programs to plan for the possibility that a cadaveric organ may become available simultaneously with a living donor transplant event. Clearly it is unacceptable to decline an available liver so that a living donor transplant can proceed, but it is similarly difficult logistically to cancel a living donor transplant due to the turmoil that it creates in the family of the donor and recipient, and the difficulty that is posed by the need to reschedule the transplant promptly. Thus, flexibility and the available capacity to staff two liver transplants at the same time will eventually be required for even medium sized liver transplant programs. In addition, in order to perform two simultaneous liver transplants it will be necessary for all the necessary equipment to be duplicated as well. This includes veno-venous bypass pumps, rapid infusion devices, retractors, and specialized instruments such as vascular clamps.

Split Liver Transplantation

In response to the shortage of livers, many transplant surgeons have proposed that the remarkable ability of the liver to regenerate means that a liver can potentially be used to transplant two recipients.(15) This technique has several variations. The left lateral segment can be removed and transplanted to a child, leaving segments III-VIII for an adult. Alternatively, the liver can be split into right and left lobes, with one recipient receiving segments I-IV and one receiving segments V-VIII, thus providing large enough grafts for two adults. In addition, the technique may be performed in vitro during the initial procurement, or ex vivo following conventional donor hepatectomy.

The in vitro technique has been popularized by programs with extensive living donor experience, since it amounts to essentially using the living donor technique on a cadaver donor. This adds very significant operative time to the donor operation, a consideration that may adversely impact organ quality, and may result in logistical difficulties at donor hospitals since the operations require significantly longer than traditional organ recovery procedures. These challenges can often be managed by appropriately informing the thoracic organ teams and the donor hospital of the time that will be required for an in vivo split procedure. The advantage of the in vivo technique is that the donor's hemostatic system can be used to control bleeding, and better hemostasis on the cut surface of the liver is thus possible. In addition, visualization of the biliary anatomy may be superior. It is also argued that overall ischemic time is less if the split is performed prior to cross-clamping.

The ex vivo technique has the advantage of being easier from a logistical point of view, in that the donor operation is no different from the standard liver recovery. It also may facilitate sharing of organs between centers, as both centers need not to be present during the split procedure. Finally, cadaveric organ donors are notoriously unstable, and adding four or more hours to the donor operation may compromise not only the liver grafts, but the kidneys and thoracic organs as well. There is currently no consensus on the best practice, with different regions of the United States and the world using each technique. The technique appears to have relatively limited applicability at present due to the fact that splitting unstable or older donors does not appear to be a wise practice. Given the advancing mean cadaver donor age across the world, the number of potentially "splitable" livers is becoming smaller and smaller.

Split liver transplantation may have a profound effect on operating room utilization, or it may have very little effect, depending on the technique used. To the extent that two organs are available from one donor, the number of needed resources will increase proportionally. Furthermore, if the two grafts are both for adults, it will be necessary for the center to have the ability to staff two liver transplants simultaneously. As described above, this may require two sets of each of the required equipment to be available. On the other hand, if the grafts go to into an adult and a child, the logistical problem may not exist as long as the pediatric and adult operating rooms are staffed independently. If the transplant center is also a major cadaveric donor center the practice of split liver transplantation may also impact donor operating room utilization if an in vivo technique is used.

Organ Donation Following Cardiac Death

The majority of organs donated today are from persons that became brain dead. Brain death is actually an uncommon method of dying, meaning that most deaths do not result in transplantable organs. The Institute of Medicine has recently issued reports approving the concept of organ donation following cardiac death (formally called "non-heart beating donation").(16) These initiatives have the potential to increase the number of available organs by capturing a larger fraction of the organs that the public are willing to donate. However, this practice has been hampered by the fact that donation following cardiac death may result in inferior outcome due to increased amounts of warm ischemia. This is particularly true for organs other than the kidney, as primary non-function of the graft is catastrophic in the case of hepatic, pulmonary, and cardiac transplantation.

Recently, investigators have described a method of utilizing ECMO (extra-corporeal membrane oxygenation) to support donors following declaration of cardiac death.(17) To date this technique has been used in controlled situations where the donor's medical team has advised withdrawal of ventilatory support due to profound central nervous system injury in patients that retain enough brain function that they do not meet brain death criteria. In this setting, investigators have successfully transplanted 12 kidneys and two livers using ECMO support and are examining the feasibility of expanding this technique to other hospitals, as well as applying the technique to uncontrolled donors in the emergency department setting.

The advantage of ECMO support is both physiologic and practical. From a physiologic standpoint, the organs are kept well perfused and oxygenated during the entire procurement process following cardiac death. In contrast, during conventional donation following cardiac death a period of time passes during which the organs remain warm as the incision is made and the organs exposed. Although cold perfusate may be used through an aortic cannula, this technique does not cool the organs rapidly. Techniques involving instilling iced saline into the peritoneum in order to cool the organs topically are cumbersome and inefficient. From a practical point of view, the ECMO support technique means that withdrawal of support can occur in the intensive care unit setting where the family can be present. The ECMO perfusion of the organs also means that the family can remain with their departed loved one to grieve without sacrificing organ quality. Another advantage is that an operating room is not utilized if withdrawal of support does not lead to cardiac death. Overall, the entire process is more palatable to all of the involved parties: ICU nursing, operating room nursing, anesthesiology, the donor family, and the donation coordinator due to the fact that nothing has to be rushed. As experience with this novel technique increases, other centers may begin utilizing this method for donation following cardiac death due to the natural advantages it has over conventional methods.

Islet Cell Transplantation

Type 1 diabetes currently affects approximately 0.5% of adults. The incidence is rising approximately 3% per year in the United States and worldwide. Islet transplantation has been proposed as a treatment for type 1 diabetes mellitus in that provision of healthy insulin producing islets should cure the disease. This hope has not been realized until recently. Of the 267 allografts transplanted between 1990 and 2000 only 12.4% have resulted in insulin independence for periods of more than one week, and only 8.2% have done so for periods of more than one year.(18) Shapiro and the group in Edmonton, Canada recently reported success in seven patients using a steroid free immunosuppression regimen, transplanting islets from multiple pancreas donors to each recipient, and using modern immunosuppression consisting of anti-IL2R antibody, tacrolimus, and sirolimus.(19) This report has led to a resurgence of interest in islet transplantation as well as an international interest in perfecting the technique. The technique, as described by Shapiro, involves instillation of the islets through a percutaneous trans-hepatic portal venous cannula by an interventional radiologist. If perfected this technique has the potential to replace whole organ pancreas grafting, a procedure done more than 1200 times per year annually in the United States. While this would have a major impact on operating room utilization, the technical and facility requirements for islet production mean that it is unlikely that islet transplantation will replace whole organ pancreas transplantation in the near future.

REFERENCES

1. Schulam PG, Kavoussi LR, Cheriff AD, Averch TD, Montgomery R, Moore RG, Ratner LE. Laparoscopic live donor nephrectomy: the initial 3 cases J Urol 1996 Jun;155(6):1857-9

2. Ratner LE, Kavoussi LR, Sroka M, Hiller J, Weber R, Schulam PG, Montgomery R. Laparoscopic assisted live donor nephrectomy--a comparison with the open approach. Transplantation. 1997 Jan 27;63(2):229-33.

3. Knoepp L. Smith M. Huey J. Mancino A. Barber H. Complication after laparoscopic donor nephrectomy: a case report and review. Transplantation. 1999 Aug 15; 68(3):449-51,

4. Wolf JS Jr. Merion RM. Leichtman AB. Campbell DA Jr. Magee JC. Punch JD. Turcotte JG. Konnak JW. Randomized controlled trial of hand-assisted laparoscopic versus open surgical live donor nephrectomy. Transplantation. 72(2):284-90, 2001 Jul 27.

5. Jacobs SC. Cho E. Dunkin BJ. Flowers JL. Schweitzer E. Cangro C. Fink J. Farney A. Philosophe B. Jarrell B. Bartlett ST. Laparoscopic live donor nephrectomy: the University of Maryland 3-year experience. Journal of Urology 2000; 164(5):1494-9.

6. Montgomery RA. Kavoussi LR. Su L. Sinkov V. Cohen C. Maley WR. Burdick JF. Markowitz J. Ratner LE. Improved recipient results after 5 years of performing laparoscopic donor nephrectomy. Transplantation Proceedings 2001; 33(1-2):1108-10.

7. Rudich SM. Marcovich R. Magee JC. Punch JD. Campbell DA. Merion RM. Konnak JW. Wolf JS. Hand-assisted laparoscopic donor nephrectomy: comparable donor/recipient outcomes, costs, and decreased convalescence as compared to open donor nephrectomy. Transplantation Proceedings. 2001; 33(1-2):1106-7.

8. Strong RW, Lynch SV, Ong TH, Matsunami H, Koido Y, Balderson GA. Successful liver transplantation from a living donor to her son. N Engl J Med 1990;322:1505-7.

9. Singer PA, Siegler M, Whitington PF, et al. Ethics of liver transplantation with living donors. N Engl J Med 1989;321:620-2.

10. Piper JB. Whitington PF. Woodle ES. Newell KA. Alonso EM. Thistlethwaite JR. Living related liver transplantation in children: a report of the first 58 recipients at the University of Chicago. Transplant International. 1994: 7 Suppl 1:S111-3.

11. Sindhi R. Rosendale J. Mundy D. Taranto S. Baliga P. Reuben A. Rajagopalan PR. Hebra A. Tagge E. Othersen HB Jr. Impact of segmental grafts on pediatric liver transplantation--a review of the United Network for Organ Sharing Scientific Registry data (1990-1996). of Pediatric Surgery. 34(1):107-10.

12. Ghobrial RM. Amersi F. Busuttil RW. Surgical advances in liver transplantation. Living related and split donors. Clinics in Liver Disease 2000; 4(3):553-65.

13. Yamaoka Y. Washida M. Honda K. Tanaka K. Mori K. Shimahara Y. Okamoto S. Ueda M. Hayashi M. Tanaka A. Liver transplantation using a right lobe graft from a living related donor. Transplantation. 1994; 57(7):1127-30.

14. Lo CM. Fan ST. Liu CL. Wei WI. Lo RJ. Lai CL. Chan JK. Ng IO. Fung A. Wong J. Adult-to-adult living donor liver transplantation using extended right lobe grafts. Annals of Surgery 1997; 226(3):261-9.

15. Busuttil RW, Goss JA. Split liver transplantation: a review. Ann Surg 1999; 229: 313-321.

16. Non-Heart Beating Organ Transplantation: Practice and Protocols. Institute of Medicine; 2000. National Academy Press, Washington, D.C.

17. Rudich SM, Arenas JD, Magee JC, Gravel MT, Chenault II RH, Kayler LK, Merion RM, Punch JD. Extracorporeal support of the non-heart beating organ donor. Transplantation, 2002 73(1):158-159.

18. Brendel M, Hering B, Schulz A, Bretzel R. International Islet Transplant Registry report. Giessen, Germany: University of Giessen, 1999:1-20.

19. Shapiro AM. Lakey JR. Ryan EA. Korbutt GS. Toth E. Warnock GL. Kneteman NM. Rajotte RV. Islet transplantation in seven patients with type 1 diabetes mellitus using a glucocorticoid-free immunosuppressive regimen. (see comments). New Engl J Med 2000. 343(4):230-8.

CHAPTER 15

UROLOGIC SURGERY

J. STUART WOLF, JR., M.D.

Although the practice of urology encompasses a variety of non-surgical components, this presentation will be restricted to the future of urologic surgery in the 21st century. Although it is likely that most of the advances in health care in the next century will be non-surgical in nature, surgical practice will advance and the need for surgery will persist. There always will be trauma, irreversible organ damage, congenital anomalies, and other disease states that medicines or other non-surgical therapy will not be able to address.(1)

The overwhelming trend in surgery is toward minimally invasive procedures foreshadowing the eventual adoption of completely non-invasive surgical therapy.(2) A century from now the overt practice of Surgery will bear only a small resemblance to that of today, but the underlying ideas will remain the same. Incising into the body has been the activity that that most explicitly distinguishes surgeons from colleagues in Internal Medicine. At a more basic level, surgery is that branch of health care where physical alteration of tissue is the primary therapeutic modality, in distinction from the pharmacological alterations that are the primary modalities in Internal Medicine. As surgery moves from manual manipulation of tissue through incisions towards energy based alteration of tissue applied extracorporeally, the overt appearance of surgery will change but the underlying principles of practice will remain.

The Appearance of Surgery in the 21st Century

Minimally invasive surgery was first integrated into routine practice by urologists, in the form of cystoscopy. Endoscopic surgery has been embraced by this specialty for over a century. Most of the genitourinary organs can be approached endoscopically.(3) Indeed, this is one of the reasons why urologists in general were somewhat slow to adopt laparoscopy. Since so much of urologic practice was already endoscopic in nature, the potential application of laparoscopy for a single surgeon was perceived to be inadequate. A few pioneering urologists were at the forefront of operative laparoscopy, in devising procedures to address cryptorchidism, but more advanced procedures such as nephrectomy (performed initially in 1990) have become popular only in the past few years. Drawing the distinction between endoscopy (use of an endoscopic through a natural body channel) and laparoscopy (use of an endoscopic in a closed body cavity), it is clear that endoscopy is fundamentally less invasive. As such, urologists will continue to strive to enhance the role of endoscopy, likely replacing laparoscopy for some procedures as new instruments and techniques are devised. For example, one might imagine that the kidney, with access to the center of the organ possible through 3 large luminal structures (main renal artery, main renal vein, and ureter) could in the future be ablated and potentially removed with endoscopic techniques. Both laparoscopy and endoscopy are steps on the journey towards completely non-invasive surgery.

Imaging

Of all the senses, it is vision that is the most critical for the surgeon. Indeed, operative laparoscopy did not expand beyond a few enthusiasts until the CCD (charge-coupled device) camera allowed display of the laparoscopic field on a monitor for the entire operative team to view.(4) Other digital image capturing devices are being considered that may improve resolution and reduce costs. "High definition television" is already enhancing video resolution. Light sources will improve to provide even more light with narrower cables. Better ways of presenting visual information will also become standard, such as heads-up displays, holographic projections, and fusion of preoperative with real time imaging. Real time imaging might include the current modalities of ultrasonography and open MRI, but also might include newer technologies that will blur the distinction between radiography and direct visual assessment. Intra-operative imaging will mature from a distinct step in the surgical procedure to an integrated component throughout the entire operation. There will be a marriage of imaging and surgical instrumentation into a single set of tools. As a urologic example, such instruments would be useful for partial nephrectomy. For renal tumors < 4 cm, or those occurring in the setting of solitary kidney or compromised renal function, partial nephrectomy may be preferable to radical (total) nephrectomy. Currently, intra-operative ultrasonography is used to delineate the margins of the mass, but then the surgical excision is performed separately. Simultaneous imaging and cutting would be more accurate and efficient. Such developments will facilitate the advancement and acceptance of minimally invasive and, eventually, completely non-invasive surgery.

Similarly, accurate preoperative imaging of the human body and its disease states has been a prerequisite to advanced minimally invasive surgery. One would not perform laparoscopic radical nephrectomy for a suspected malignancy without accurate imaging of the kidney and abdominal contents. For minimally invasive surgery to progress towards non-invasive surgery, there first will have to be improvements in imaging. There will be growth in two areas: improvement on existing technology and development of new imaging modalities. With regard to the former, advances in the resolution and bandwidth of ultrasonography and magnetic resonance imaging will provide real time imaging and also more accurate preoperative depiction of anatomical abnormalities, without exposure to ionizing radiation. The fusion of anatomical and functional imaging, such as MRI together with PET scanning, will allow more accurate preoperative determination of disease and obviate the need for exploratory surgery.

The addition of new imaging modalities will expand the promise even more. Optical coherence tomography is such a technique, one that will provide for virtual histological sampling of intact tissue and render actual tissue biopsy unnecessary. Ultrasonographic measurement of elasticity, which allows microscopic "palpation" of deep structures, is another potentially useful modality; researchers have already demonstrated accurate imaging of the prostate with this technique. Other technologies, used to accurately assess microscopic blood flow, metabolism, and numerous additional tissue characteristics, might be applied to improve preoperative diagnosis.

New Instrumentation

The creation of new instruments and surgical techniques has been integral to the development of minimally invasive surgery. The Seldinger technique, balloon dilators, lasers, biologic glues, and ultrasonic coagulation are but a few of the important advances in this regard. The traditional surgical instrumentation of a forceps and scissors are still useful and versatile, but need to be improved for the laparoscopic or other minimally invasive setting. The limitation of moving a long narrow device with a handle on one end and an effector on the other, rotating about a fixed point on the abdominal wall, must be surpassed. Simple articulation, currently available on only a few devices, will be replaced by end effectors with multiple degrees of freedom, now incorporated into the instruments for the da Vinci robotic system (Intuitive Surgical). For procedures performed in a limited space, such as laparoscopic radical prostatectomy with the challenging anastomosis created at the very apex of the pelvis, articulation with multiple degrees of freedom is much more effective than a straight instrument. Improvements in the sense of touch (haptic feedback) provided by hand-held instruments will be a welcome development.

In addition, the interface between the human hand and the end effector will be improved, perhaps with something resembling the "data glove" now seen in some virtual reality simulators. This would minimize fatigue, shorten the "learning curve," and allow the surgeon to concentrate on the task at hand rather than physical manipulation of the instruments. Instruments will be multifunctional, providing hemostasis, cutting, and dissecting, as well as palpation, imaging, or other diagnostic modalities, all in one device. Miniaturization and creation of additional flexible instruments that can be used endoscopically are also anticipated.

Nano-instrumentation

Nanotechnology conceptually meshes with minimally invasive surgery. With very small electromechanical tools and devices, minimally invasive surgery could move beyond mere approximation of open surgical techniques into the realm of the new and improved surgical procedures. Nano-instruments might be affixed to the effector end of laparoscopic instruments to assist in tissue identification or dissection.

Even further in the future, one can envision freely mobile nano-instruments, perhaps deployed laparoscopically at the site of disease or "set free" into natural body channels, that might identify, isolate, and treat disease.

Robotics

It now seems certain that robots will play a major role in the evolution of minimally invasive surgery.(5,6) Robots allow the surgeon more complete control of the operative situation, reduce hand tremor, and provide movement scaling. Fatigue of the surgeon is minimized, and operative techniques can be more standardized. Robots also are part of the enormous system that will be required to perform telesurgical procedures (see below). Robots to hold the laparoscope, and to assist with orthopedic and neurosurgical procedures, are well accepted. The most advanced operative robot currently available is the da Vinci system (Intuitive Surgical). In urology, use of the robot for nephrectomy, adrenalectomy, and pyeloplasty have been reported — but the most common use has been for radical prostatectomy.(7-9) Proponents of the robot argue that it reduces fatigue, simplifies some complex steps of the procedure, and improves outcome owing to improved vision and camera stabilization. In truth, there are still major deficiencies that limit the da Vinci robots utility, and the overall balance of advantages and disadvantages for radical prostatectomy is uncertain. The most significant limitation is lack of the sense of touch (haptic feedback). It appears that this robot enhances surgical technique beyond that of a skilled laparoscopic surgeon only in the setting of fine detail work that can be performed under visual control, such as laparoscopic suturing. Future robots, with haptic feedback and other sensing modalities, will undoubtedly be superior to direct manual surgery.

Tissue Sensors

Implicit in the discussion above regarding new instrumentation and robotics is the need for improved direct sensing of the tissues upon which we are operating. Haptic feedback and the ultrasonographic measurement of elasticity (to assess tissue stiffness, i.e. "virtual palpation") have been mentioned, but there are other tissue characteristics that could be sensed by the end effector of the instrument. Detection of subtle temperature differences, histological composition, and vascularity might be some of the distinctions that we could someday use in real time to optimize surgical procedures.

Bioinformatics

The emerging field of bioinformatics will be relied upon to analyze and interpret the huge amount of data generated from genomics and other large-scale tissue studies. The information technology thus developed could be logically applied to surgical informatics problems such as video processing, control of robots, and analysis of information from new imaging and tissue-sensing instruments.

Tissue Approximation

Suturing remains the most versatile of our tissue approximation methods. Sutures, however, create ischemia, invoke a foreign body response, and can be a nidus for infection. One would anticipate that this method of tissue approximation, in use for thousands of years, will not continue to hold prominence through the next century. Alternative techniques such as staples, tissue glue, and laser welding are already with us, and have their place for a specific few applications. In Urology, laparoscopic staplers provide rapid tissue and vascular control in many situations, tissue glue is used by many surgeons for hemostasis during laparoscopic partial nephrectomy, and laser welding is reported to reduce the fistula rate associated with hypospadias repair. Overall, however, these techniques are limited by their poor adaptation to tissue and low tolerance for misapplication. In order to advance minimally invasive reconstructive procedures, improved methods of tissue approximation will need to be developed.

Energy-based Therapy

Physical alteration of tissue rather than actual resection has already been introduced in a variety of settings. In urology, cryoablation of prostate cancer and renal tumors has been widely reported. Interstitial radiofrequency coagulation has been used for many years in the prostate, and is now being applied to renal tumors in some centers. Both of these technologies, as well as other energy-based modalities, are applicable to laparoscopic and "needle invasive" procedures. The only currently available energy-based therapy that offers the potential for completely extracorporeal (non invasive) therapy is HIFU (high intensity focused ultrasound). Urologically, HIFU has been applied in a limited setting to the prostate, bladder, and kidney. Skin burns and focal distance limit the current single transducer devices, but future devices, likely incorporating a phased array of numerous piezoelectric elements, might overcome these problems. In order for minimally invasive surgery to progress, we must accept energy-based ablation of tissue rather than physical resection, and must be open to the establishment of new treatment paradigms involving extracorporeal application of energy. The positive experience of urologists with extracorporeal shockwave lithotripsy for urinary calculi, one of the first widespread applications of extracorporeal therapy in surgery, will facilitate this acceptance.

Minimally Invasive Delivery of Targeted Agents

Soluble therapy targeted to specific malignancies will become more commonplace. Targeting can be achieved through antigenic matching or other techniques. The targeted agent might be immunologic, pharmacologic, anti-angiogenic, or related to a number of cytokines. The optimal agents would deliver therapeutic activity to the target without systemic adverse effects even during systemic administration.

It is possible that physical delivery of therapy to the target site, either by endoscopy or laparoscopy, would enhance the activity of some of these agents. We must "think outside the box" in terms of expanding surgery to include such techniques.

Tissue Engineering

Although our current abilities to transplant organs and to create functional approximations of new organs (neobladders, buccal mucosal grafts for urethral stricture disease, etc.) have improved the lives of thousands of patients, progress has come at a price. Morbidity and risk to another individual in the case of live organ donation, and to the donor tissue site in the case of autologous reconstruction, are not insignificant. There are great expectations for the techniques of tissue engineering in this regard. The ability to routinely synthesize relatively simple biologic structures such as connective tissues might be expected in the next few years. Using porous synthetic scaffolds, cell engineering techniques such as viral transfection, and analysis of the human genome, more complex organs might well be created "at the bench" for surgical placement in diseased individuals, thereby reducing the risk to donating individuals and donor tissue sites.

Moreover, the current reconstructive procedures do not always provide the exact functional equivalent of the organ being replaced. Artificial organs that are structural replicates of the original healthy organ should duplicate function as well. Such artificial organs will be created with the minimally invasive approach to implantation in mind, such that the end result will be superior organ replacements or reconstructions with minimized peri-operative morbidity.

Telemedicine

Telemedicine is a broad term describing the transmission of video or still images between distant sites for the purpose of health care. The simplest form is teleconsultation, which involves the transmission of images from a remote site to a physician who reports findings and conclusions back to that site.(10) The other end of the spectrum is telesurgery, which involves active control of surgical instruments by a surgeon from a remote site. Urologists at Johns Hopkins University have been at the forefront of telesurgery, with the report of transatlantic control of a videolaparoscope and electrocautery during laparoscopic adrenalectomy, nephrectomy, and varicocelectomy (surgeon in Baltimore, and patients in Innsbruck, Bangkok, and Singapore, respectively) in 1998. Although the potential for telesurgery is exciting with regards to surgical procedures done in remote locations (battlefield, outer space, etc.), it is likely that the greatest utility of telemedicine will be for teleproctoring and telementoring. The former is the real time observation and evaluation of a surgeon's performance by an expert at a remote location. This requires only one-way communication in real time. Telementoring, the two-way transmission of video and audio information for real time feedback and instruction, is a more exciting possibility.

Telementoring will likely play a larger role in surgical training in the future. We are all familiar with the "long" learning curve of many minimally invasive procedures. With the expectation that most or all urologists will perform advanced minimally invasive procedures in the future, the potential risk to patients imposed by every single one of them passing through a "long" learning curve is unacceptable. We must provide more expert training. The initial experiences with telementoring have revealed that this is an effective way to impart surgical knowledge, second only to direct face-to-face contact between the mentor and student in the operating room. Although teaching in person works well for a residency program, it is not feasible for widespread promulgation of new techniques to physicians already in practice. Telementoring offers an excellent substitute that will markedly enhance the training of practicing physicians.

Training Techniques

In order to train urologic surgeons to perform new procedures a variety of new educational techniques will be needed. Computer-generated virtual reality surgery, a realistic three-dimensional representation of a surgical procedure that provides interaction and feedback, will likely play a large role in training and the planning of surgical procedures. Operations will be performed in a virtual reality simulator before a patient is exposed to risk. In addition, operating rooms will be wired for broadband communications to share real-time audio and video between sites. One could envision a program whereby trainees and surgeons in practice could routinely log on to any number of published live operations, or download the files from an archive of procedures, for training purposes

Incorporation of Advances into Environment Design

All of the aforementioned advances require consideration when creating the operating room of the future. Surgeons will need to be creative in moving from current concepts in order to realize the potential for combining advances into an environment conducive to the best possible surgery. Part radiology suite, part intensive care unit, part lecture hall, and part operating room, the surgical suite of the future must be wired for broadband audio and video transmission. The current wasteful practice of rolling instruments in and out of the room, with ancillary staff members spending a considerable one of time setting up and breaking down, needs to be replaced. Because these rooms likely carry a great capital expense, strategies for maximizing usage (extended work hours, alternate patient preparation and recovery protocols, etc) must be considered. Already there are excellent endoscopic operating rooms that used booms, fixed instrumentation, and complete hardwiring for video and audio. Continued progress must be made in this regard, with the focus of maximizing efficiency, safety, and training during the delivery of surgical care.

Conclusion

The game of prediction is fraught with difficulty. Even with only a few specific predictions, surely many will prove inaccurate. The path that urologic surgery will take in the transition from open surgical procedures to minimally invasive surgery to non-invasive therapy will undoubtedly be bumpy, with more than a few missteps and injuries along the way. However, the close of the 21st century will see a transformed urologic surgical practice that provides far greater enhancement of patients' lives and far less iatrogenic morbidity than is currently possible.

REFERENCES

1. Griffith LG and Grodzinsky AJ: Advances in Biomedical Engineering. JAMA 285: 556 - 561, 2001.

2. Hunter JG: Minimally invasive surgery: the new frontier. World J, Surg. 23: 422 - 424, 1999.

3. Kakizoe T: Urologic oncology in the twenty-first century. World J. Surg. 24: 1167 - 1171, 2000.

4. Kourambas J and Preminger GM: Advances in camera, video, and imaging technologies in laparoscopy. Urol Clin North Am. 28: 5 - 14, 2001.

5. Link RE, Schulam PG and Kavoussi LR: Telesurgery. Remote monitoring and assistance during laparoscopy. Urol Clin North Am. 28: 177 - 188, 2001.

6. Mack MJ: Minimally invasive and robotic surgery. JAMA 285: 568 - 572, 2001.

7. Matsuda T, Kawakita M and Terachi T: Future of Urologic laparoscopy. World J. Surg. 24: 1172 - 1175, 2000.

8. McConnell JD: The development of urology in the 21st century. BJU International 88 (Suppl. 2): 2 - 6, 2001.

9. Shah J, Mackay S, Rockall T, Vale J and Darzi A: Urorobotic: robots in Urology. BJU International 88: 313 - 320, 2001.

10. Tempany CMC and McNeil BJ: Advances in Biomedical Imaging. JAMA 285: 562 - 567, 2001.

CHAPTER 16

VASCULAR SURGERY

MATTHEW J. EAGLETON, M.D., GILBERT R. UPCHURCH, JR., M.D.

The United States population is aging at an unprecedented rate. Between 2010 and 2030, the population over the age of 65 years will increase by 75% due to aging baby boomers. During this same period, the population younger than 65 years will decrease by 3%.(1) Based on these estimates, it is projected that the number of peripheral vascular operative interventions required will increase from 232 to 313 procedures per 100,000 persons. This translates into greater than 1,020,000 vascular operations in the year 2020.(2) Therefore, there is little doubt that the care given to patients with peripheral vascular disease (PVD) both in and out of the operating room will need to radically change over the next 20 years.

Scientific Advances

While it is unlikely that atherosclerosis and other vascular diseases will be eradicated, preventative medical care will help to decrease the surgical burden incurred with the aging population. Prophylactic monitoring and treatment of patients genetically prone to vascular disease will be widespread. Noninvasive technology, such as measuring the carotid artery intima media thickness, will aid in the early diagnosis of atherosclerosis prior to clinical manifestations and will dictate who is placed on aggressive lipid-lowering and antihypertensive agents prophylactically.(Figure 1) In addition, genetic codes will be used to screen for various vascular diseases, similar to colonoscopy and stool guaiacs for early detection of colon cancer.

Along with the development of new screening tools, advances in vascular biology will lead to the discovery of pharmacologic and genetic therapies that prevent or retard atherosclerosis, aneurysmal disease and intimal hyperplasia. Many of these new therapies will be delivered using standard oral or parenteral routes. However, others will require endovascular or transluminal delivery in order to assure that they are administered at high concentrations to specific vascular beds. The investigational use of gene therapy using recombinant deoxyribonucleic acid (DNA) or proteins to treat non-reconstructible peripheral arterial occlusive disease will expand. While presently injected intramuscularly, as safety profiles are improved, direct intra-arterial delivery of recombinant gene or protein constructs will be performed with increased efficacy.

Vascular surgery is already using less invasive, more cost effective technology. For example, it was once considered radical and unsafe to perform carotid endarterectomy (CEA) without first obtaining a diagnostic invasive angiogram. Presently,

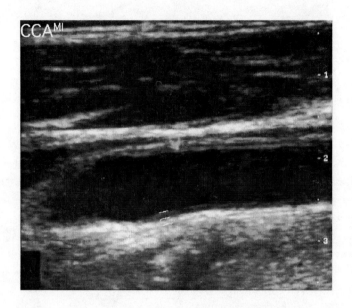

Figure 16-1

Less invasive tests, such as carotid artery intima/media thickness determined by duplex ultrasonography, will be used to diagnose subtle atherosclerosis prior to the manifestation of symptoms. Note no gross disease in asymptomatic 40-year-old male. I – intima, M – media, CCA – common carotid artery

preoperative arteriography is considered obsolete and potentially dangerous due to the small antecedent risk of stroke following an arteriogram. Currently, non-invasive duplex ultrasonography, at a fraction of the cost of arteriography, is the only diagnostic study performed prior to CEA. For a number of other vascular procedures, the preoperative workup has been altered substantially to lessen both the invasive nature and the risks. Patients now routinely undergo endovascular abdominal aortic aneurysm (AAA) repair following a non-invasive CT scan with three-dimensional (3-D) reconstructions as the only diagnostic study performed prior to AAA repair. (Figure 2) However, today's standard 3-D CT scanner does expose the patient to the risk of intravenous nephrotoxic iodinated contrast. In the future, electron beam CT scanners will not require iodinated contrast and will be used diagnostically and therapeutically to guide invasive and endoluminal therapy.

The use of catheter-based techniques to treat atherosclerotic and aneurysmal vascular disease will escalate over the next 20 years. As many as 50% of lesions once thought to be amenable only to surgery will be treated transluminally in the future.3 It should be noted that the efficacy and safety of many of these less invasive treatments have not been scientifically validated against standard surgical therapy. However, both the treating physician and the vascular patient are often willing to trade inferior patency and effectiveness for decreased morbidity, reduced lengths of stay and possibly lower hospital and health care costs.

Peripheral Arterial Interventions

Since the 1960s when Dotter introduced the concept of intravascular interventions, there has been tremendous progress in the evolution of endovascular therapy. Percutaneous transluminal angioplasty (PTA) with stenting is presently used to treat occlusive disease in a variety of locations. When used for the common iliac artery (CIA) it has been associated with low morbidity and mortality and 5-year patency rates approaching that of conventional aortofemoral bypass. In addition, patients

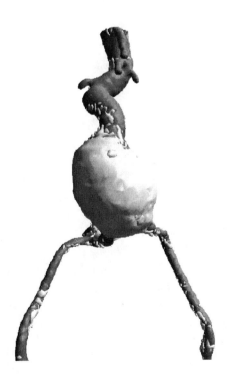

Figure 16-2

Three-dimensional CT scan of aorta performed as the only diagnostic test prior to endovascular AAA repair allows for diameter determination of aortic neck and iliac arteries.

who undergo PTA with stenting of the CIA sustain a significant quality of life improvement.(4, 5) PTA with stenting is also technically successful in the external iliac artery, but has inferior long-term patency results compared with the common iliac artery.(6) However, endovascular treatment of more distal peripheral vascular occlusive disease has not been as successful. A meta-analysis of PTA with stenting for femoropopliteal arterial occlusive disease revealed three year patency rates of 60%.(7) This is clearly lower than reported patency rates for femoral to distal artery bypasses using an autogenous venous conduit.

PTA with stenting is not limited to the pelvic and lower extremity arteries, but is being applied to the renal and visceral arteries with excellent technical success.(8,9) The results of mesenteric artery stenting for chronic ischemia in particular appear to be comparable to conventional surgery with regards to morbidity, mortality, and recurrent stenosis. Primary stenting of the mesenteric vessels has also been associated with an earlier return of gastrointestinal symptoms.(10)

Another transluminal procedure under investigation is carotid artery stenting. This is presently indicated in patients with significant cerebrovascular occlusive disease who have excessive risk for surgery and anesthesia, early post-CEA restenosis secondary to intimal hyperplasia, or radiation-induced stenosis. While early results suggest that carotid artery stenting can be performed technically,(11) as yet, no randomized, prospective clinical trial has established its safety and long-term prevention of stroke compared to conventional CEA, which remains the gold standard. Ongoing multicenter trials comparing carotid artery stenting and CEA will better define the indications for and results of carotid artery stenting. However, the fact that carotid artery stenting is being performed, prior to the development of adequate rescue devices to prevent atherosclerotic debris from causing a stroke, may doom this technology.

One of the major limitations of stent placement, regardless of anatomic location of the lesion being treated, is restenosis. Current approaches used to prevent stent restenosis come from research performed primarily in the coronary circulation. A promising area of research is the use of radiation to prevent restenosis. Initial results from a prospective, randomized, controlled trial with brachytherapy, using a beta-emitter on coronary arteries following balloon angioplasty and stent placement, showed significantly lower restenosis rates in patients receiving radiation.(12) Future applications of brachytherapy may lead to the placement of radioactive stents that continuously supply a low level of radiation to the surrounding vessel, thereby potentially reducing restenosis rates.

To date, many pharmacologic approaches to prevent restenosis have failed; primarily due to an inability to attain intravascular therapeutic drug levels.(13) An alternative to using intravascular medications or radiation involves chemically-treated stents that may provide higher local levels of various pharmacologic agents. In human coronary arteries, the placement of stents coated with sirolimus, a potent immunosuppressive agent that inhibits the proliferation of smooth muscle cells, has been investigated.(14) Initial evaluation, by intravascular ultrasound and coronary angiography, documented minimal neointimal hyperplasia and no in-stent or edge restenosis at a mean of follow-up of 8 months. The development of these pharmacologically "enhanced" stents to prevent restenosis might improve results with stenting in certain vascular beds, such as the femoral and popliteal arteries.

New Operative Approaches

Many vascular patients requiring surgery are elderly, with significant comorbidities, and are therefore unable to tolerate the excessive metabolic demands incurred with traditional open surgery. A less invasive therapeutic treatment may also not be an option. Vascular surgery has responded to this challenge by developing new modalities to treat vascular disease, including applications of laparoscopy/endoscopy.

Laparoscopy

General Surgery has been altered forever by the use of laparoscopy, as operations such as cholecystectomy and Nissen fundoplication are rarely performed now using open techniques. Laparoscopy has lead to shortened hospital stays and a quicker return to routine daily activities in the perioperative period. Although vascular surgery has been slow to adopt laparoscopy, recent results suggest that it may play a larger role in the vascular practice of the future. For example, wound complications following traditional open saphenous vein harvest remain a large source of morbidity and increased cost following lower extremity revascularization.(15,16) In an attempt to reduce the incidence of wound complications, endoscopic techniques for saphenous vein harvest are being employed,(17) with endoscopic-guided clipping of saphenous vein side branches through small incisions, followed by an in situ bypass. Suggs has suggested that this modality leads to a significantly lower number of wound complications, as well as shorter hospital stays compared to patients undergoing standard vein harvest techniques, yet provides similar graft patencies.(18)

Endoscopic techniques are also being used for division of incompetent venous perforators to aid in the treatment of venous stasis ulcers caused by venous insufficiency. This procedure involves the placement of endoscopic ports through two small incisions in the subfascial plane, which is expanded with carbon dioxide.(19) Then, medial perforating veins are clipped and divided. This technique is significantly less invasive than the classic Linton procedure with early and mid-term results from the North American Subfascial Endoscopic Perforator Surgery (SEPS) registry suggesting it is safe and effective in decreasing the symptoms of chronic venous insufficiency, leading to higher rates of venous stasis ulcer healing.(20,21)

Importantly, the frequency of early complications after SEPS is significantly less than after open surgery.

Conventional aortic procedures are also being performed using laparoscopic-assisted techniques. Din and colleagues performed the first documented laparoscopic-assisted aortobifemoral bypass graft in humans.(22) Since the original description, several series have reported various techniques for performing technically successful laparoscopic-assisted aorto-bifemoral bypass. Transperitoneal and retroperitoneal exposure, as well as hand-assisted laparoscopic surgery has been described for aortoiliac occlusive disease (AIOD).(23-27) To date, most operations have involved laparoscopic exposure of the aorta with a conventional sutured end to side graft to aorta anastomosis. Others have utilized a less invasive endosuture technique.

In the future, laparoscopic aortic surgery will not be limited to AIOD. In fact, laparoscopic-assisted AAA repair has also been described.(28-32) This procedure involves either laparoscopic-assisted aneurysm surgery or aneurysm exclusion. A single report has described a total laparoscopic endoaneurysmorrhaphy.(33) As with laparoscopic aortobifemoral bypass, these cases have been associated with shorter hospital stays and less morbidity.

These preliminary series suggest that laparoscopic-assisted aortic surgery is feasible and safe regardless of the method used. The approach is associated with earlier postoperative ambulation, less need for analgesia and decreased hospital length of stay. While future procedures may likely utilize a completely laparoscopic approach, it is also possible that new techniques will merely modify current ones. New endosuturing techniques which allow graft to vessel anastomoses to be performed more easily and quicker are expected by 2020.(34)

Endovascular Abdominal Aortic Aneurysm Repair

An alternative to laparoscopic aortic aneurysm repair is endovascular aortic stent grafting. (Figure 3) Endovascular repair of AAAs is associated with significantly less intraoperative hemodynamic and metabolic stress than conventional open AAA surgery (35) leading to decreased morbidity.(36-37) Because of this, many patients who are not candidates for conventional aortic surgery may tolerate aortic endografting. The future success of this approach will depend on the development of lower profile grafts with broader applications, as many women are excluded from endografting because of the small diameter of their iliac arteries. AAA exclusion by endografting can also result in an endoleak, which occurs when blood flow remains in the aneurysm sac. When this occurs, the aneurysm is not excluded and the patient is still at risk for rupture. Improved identification and treatment of endoleaks must occur in the future, as the incidence of endoleaks after 3 to 4 years is between 10-30%.(38) The long-term effect of persistent endoleaks without aneurysm enlargement is unknown, as is the long-term durability of endografts materials.

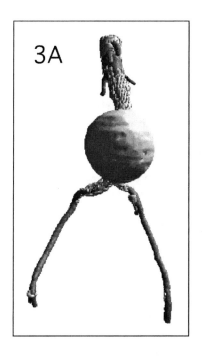
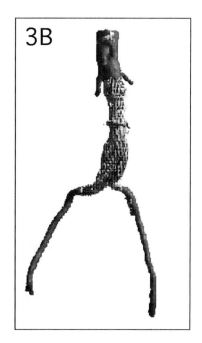

Figure 16-3

Three-dimensional CT scan of aortic endograft in the presence (A) and absence (B) of aortic thrombus showing infrarenal bifurcated endograft excluding a large AAA.

Currently, endografting is used primarily in the treatment of infrarenal AAAs. However, in the future, endografting of thoracoabdominal aortic aneurysms (TAAA) involving the renal and visceral circulation will be possible. Early experience with endoluminal aortic grafting of aneurysms with renal and mesenteric artery involvement has been technically successful.(Figure 4) These complicated endografts allow for preservation of arterial blood flow to the renal and visceral vessels through fenestrations and short branches off of the main endograft.(39-42) Continued development of this technique could eventually significantly reduce the excessive morbidity and mortality associated with TAAA repair.

Endovascular repair of ruptured AAAs may also provide an opportunity to improve the outcome from this devastating complication that has not seen an improvement in mortality over the past 20 years. Preliminary results with endovascular repair of ruptured AAAs suggest it is feasible and may lower the mortality of conventional open repair.(43,44)

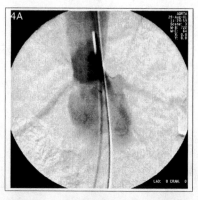

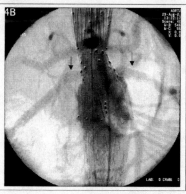

Figure 16-4

Preoperative (A) and postoperative arteriogram (B) in a patient with a pararenal aortic aneurysm. The Cook® Zenith endovascular fenestrated graft was placed following bilateral renal artery stenting (Arrows). (Photographs furnished by Dr. Roy Greenburg, Cleveland Clinic)

Telemedicine, Telepresence Surgery, and Robotics

Along with the use of laparoscopy and endovascular technologies, vascular surgery will use telemedicine, telepresence surgery, and robotics. To date, telemedicine has been limited to supplying diagnostic and consultative services to remote areas.45 Teleoperation (control of remote instruments by an operator manipulating levers) and telepresence (control of remote instruments with multisensory input allowing for tactile, audio, and visual cues) are currently in development.(46) Tissue dissection, vessel manipulation, and suturing using these techniques are being tested in preclinical trials, and have demonstrated a precision equal to that of conventional techniques.(47) Further work has shown that complex 3-D manipulations are possible, including microsurgical vascular anastomoses.(48,49) The clinical application of this technology, using microinstruments through small ports, is broad ranging and will allow for care in areas where surgical specialists are not available. Similar technology using surgical robotic systems is being used in coronary artery bypass grafting and allows closed-chest coronary artery bypass surgery without the need for cardiopulmonary bypass.(50)

Converting the Vascular Operating Room to an Endovascular Suite

While the future vascular operating room (OR) will need to support conventional vascular surgical procedures, it will also need to contain the equipment required to perform endoscopic/laparoscopic and endovascular procedures. Therefore, a vascular therapeutics suite (VTS) will be needed that will allow these less invasive procedures to be performed in conjunction with conventional open vascular surgery. In the future, a patient with iliac artery stenosis will have stent placement prior to distal lower extremity revascularization performed simultaneously in the VTS and based on a noninvasive preoperative work-up. The VTS will allow immediate diagnosis and correction of suboptimal results, the treatment of previously unrecognized or unexpected lesions, and multiple interventions in a single setting.(51)

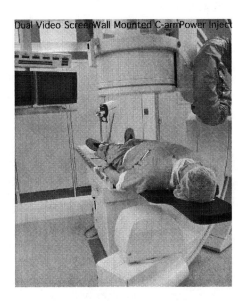

Figure 16-5

Present endovascular suite at the Ann Arbor Veterans Affairs Hospital with a wall-mounted C-arm, power injector, radiolucent table and dual video screen.

The transformation of the present OR into a VTS has already begun in many centers.(Figure 5) While current ORs may accommodate makeshift portable video equipment, the full conversion into a VTS requires capital investment, increased space, and planning. The largest physical addition to the operating room is radiographic equipment. While present day C-arm units provide room to room mobility, the image quality, reliability, and reproducibility of fixed or wall-mounted systems is far superior.(52,53) However, these fixed systems require special construction and are quite costly. Special operating tables are also required. Movable, radiolucent tables provide the best visualization during endovascular procedures, but may be cumbersome during conventional operations. In addition, the trend away from ionizing radiation requires that the VTS contain an intraoperative intravascular ultrasound machine. The VTS will be stocked with a wide variety of disposable supplies and costly peripherals, such as angiographic sheaths, catheters, guidewires, angioplasty balloons, stents, and stent grafts. The VTS must also allow the application of telepresence surgery. While anesthetic equipment and personnel may still be present, the VTS may not require presence of a vascular surgeon, or any surgeon for that matter. In fact, the surgeon may be in an adjacent control room or even at a remote location. Optimization of the human-computer interface will vastly improve the application of this technology.(48)

The Vascular Patient Caregiver

With all of this developing technology, who will be providing care for the patient with vascular disease in the year 2020? The present paradigm has the vascular surgeon managing most all peripheral vascular needs, including traditionally non-operative diseases such as venous stasis ulcers, Raynaud's disease, and claudication. In the future, it is unclear whether this will continue. At present, vascular surgery as a discipline is inadequately equipped to take care of the nearly 76 million Medicare beneficiaries who will be greater than 65 years of age by the year 2030.(54) With increasing work force demands, either the number of vascular surgeons trained must increase or another group of physicians will need to become more involved in the care of patients with peripheral vascular disease (PVD). Cardiologists, with numbers far exceeding that of vascular surgery and interventional radiology, may assume the responsibility for patients with peripheral vascular disease primarily. Cardiologists have ready access to patients with PVD and also have the prerequisite catheter-based skills required to treat many of the peripheral vascular lesions. It is possible that the workforce paradigm will shift, with cardiologists playing a significantly larger role and interventional radiologists, who are primarily procedure-oriented, ceasing to be involved in the care of vascular patients.(Figure 6) This latter paradigm already exists for patients requiring coronary care.

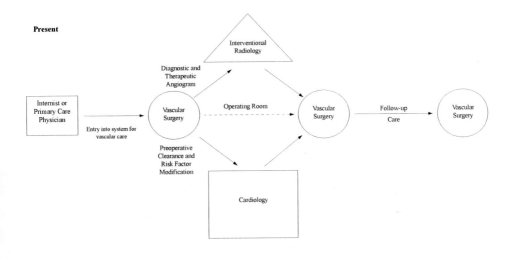

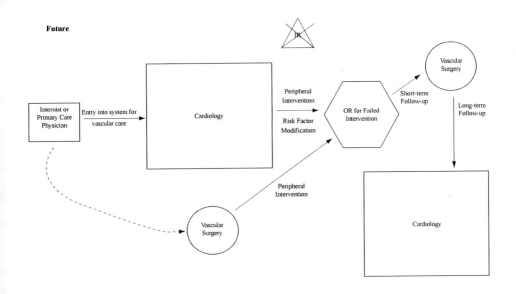

Figure 16-6

Present and future paradigm for care of the patient with vascular disease.

The Vascular Surgery Workforce

Regardless of the paradigm in place, more vascular surgeons with both open and interventional skills will be required. Hence, work force issues must be addressed in the not so distant future or patients with vascular disease will suffer. As indicated, the massive increase in the number of vascular procedures needed by 2020 will be accompanied by an inadequate supply of skilled vascular surgeons. Outcomes-based research will verify that those who are trained to perform vascular surgery and who perform it more often have lower mortalities. Similar to present-day cardiac surgery, the technologic advances and superior training required will result in vascular surgery no longer being practiced by general surgeons, who now perform close to 50% of vascular operations.

Falling reimbursement rates will also negatively impact the future of vascular care if allowed to continue. Current reimbursement rates have had an impact on surgical therapy following the Balanced Budget Act which led to an approximately 5% per year decline in Medicare reimbursement rates over the last 5 years. This can be readily seen in cases where amputation or limb salvage procedures are options. More reasonable financial reimbursement and a decreased operative time for an amputation make this barbaric operation the primary surgical option in some vascular practices compared to limb salvage surgery, which is poorly reimbursed for the extensive time spent in the operating room. Other such examples exist in the present environment. Angioplasty and iliac artery stenting are procedures mostly performed by a non-surgeon interventionalist, yet are reimbursed similar to a femoral artery to distal tibial artery bypass that may take 4 to 6 hours. These incongruities in reimbursement rates will need to be addressed so that treatment will not be dictated by reimbursement rates. Clinical common sense must prevail with outcome rather than ease of treatment and physician reimbursement dictating patient therapy. Predictably, reimbursement for skilled vascular surgeons will increase based on the excessive demand and the limited supply of surgeons who perform open surgical procedures.

Vascular Surgery as a Guide in the Days of Web-based Medicine

New technology and imaging capabilities, as well as the ever-expanding web, will influence greatly the way patients with vascular disease seek medical and surgical care. The options available to patients with vascular disease will be overwhelming to many. The key to being an outstanding vascular surgeon will be recognizing that these developing technologies and medical breakthroughs are merely tools. Superior technical skill and compassion will still be the cornerstone of the profession. In the future, helping patients to determine which options are most appropriate will become more critical, as the possibilities for treatment will be unlimited.

Acknowledgments

The authors would like to thank Ms. Shannon Proctor for her secretarial assistance.

REFERENCES

1. Stanley JC, Barnes RW, Ernst CB, Hertzer NR, Mannick JA, et al. Vascular surgery in the United States: Workforce issues. Report of the Society for Vascular Surgery and the International Society for Cardiovascular Surgery, North American Chapter, Committee on Workforce issues. J Vasc Surg 1996; 23:172-81.

2. Stanley JC. Presidential address: The American Board of Vascular Surgery. J Vasc Surg 1998; 27:195-202.

3. Veith FJ. The Society for Vascular Surgery: A look at the future. J Vasc Surg 1996; 24:144-47.

4. Tegtmeyer C, Hardwell G, Selby B, Robertson R, Kron I, Tribble C. Results and complications of angioplasty in aortoiliac disease. Circulation (Suppl. I) 83:53;1991.

5. Bosch JL, van der Graff Y, Hunink MGM. Health-related quality of life after angioplasty and stent placement in patients with iliac artery occlusive disease: results of a randomized controlled clinical trial. Circulation 1999; 99:3155-60.

6. Lee ES, Steenson CC, Trimble KE, Caldwell MP, Kuskowski MA, Santilli SM. Comparing patency rates between external iliac and common iliac artery stents. J Vasc Surg 2000; 31:889-94.

7. Muradin GSR, Bosch JL, Stijnen T, Hunink MGM. Balloon dilation and stent implantation for treatment of femoropopliteal arterial disease: meta-analysis. Radiology 2001; 221:137-45.

8. Blum U, Bernd K, Flugel P, Gabelmann A, Lehnert T, Buitrago-Tellez C, Schollmeyer P, and Langer M. Treatment of ostial renal-artery stenoses with vascular endoprostheses after unsuccessful balloon angioplasty. N Engl J Med 1997; 336:459-65.

9. Eldrup-Jorgensen J, Harvey HR, Sampson LN, Amberson SM, Bredenberg CE. Should percutaneous transluminal renal artery angioplasty be applied to ostial renal artery atherosclerosis? J Vasc Surg 1995; 21:909-15.

10. Kasirajan K, O'Hara PJ, Gray BH, Hertzer NR, Clair DG, Greenberg RK, Krajewski LP, Beven EG, Ouriel K. Chronic mesenteric ischemia: open surgery versus percutaneous angioplasty and stenting. J Vasc Surg 2001; 33:63-71.

11. Roubin GS, New G, Iyer SS, Vitek JJ, Al-Mubarak N, Liu MW, Yadav J, Gomez C, Kunts RE. Immediate and late clinical outcomes of carotid artery stenting in patients with symptomatic and asymptomatic carotid artery stenosis. Circulation 2001; 103:532-537.

12. Raizner AE, Oesterle SN, Waksman R, Serruys PW, Colombo A, Lim YL, Yeung AC, van der Giessen WJ, Vandertie L, Chiu JK, White LR, Fitzgerald PJ, Kaluza GL, Alie NM. Inhibition of restenosis with B-emitting radiotherapy. Report of the proliferation reduction with vascular energy trial (PREVENT). Circulation 2000; 102:951-958.

13. Lafont A, Faxon D. Why do animal models of post-angioplasty restenosis sometimes poorly predict the outcome of clinical trials? Cardiovasc Res 1998; 39:50-9.

14. Sousa JE, Costa MA, Abizaid A, Abizaid AS, Feres F, Pinto IMF, et al. Lack of neointimal proliferation after implantation of sirolimus-coated stents in human coronary arteries. A quantitative coronary angiography and three-dimensional intravascular ultrasound study. Circulation 2001; 103:192-195.

15. Schwartz ME, Harrington EB, Schanzer H. Wound complications after in situ bypass. J Vasc Surg 1988; 7:802-7.

16. Kent KC, Bartek S, Kuntz KM, Anninos E, Skillman JJ. Prospective study of wound complications in continuous infrainguinal incisions after lower limb arterial reconstruction: incidence, risk factors, and cost. Surgery 1996; 119:378-83.

17. Jordan WD, Voellinger DC, Schroeder PT, McDowell HA. Video-assisted saphenous vein harvest: The evolution of a new technique. J Vasc Surg 1997; 26:405-14.

18. Suggs WD, Sanchez LA, Woo DA, Lipsitz EC, Ohki T, Veith FJ. Endoscopically assisted in situ lower extremity bypass graft: A preliminary report of a new minimally invasive technique. J Vasc Surg 2001; 34:668-72.

19. Gloviczki P, Cambria RA, Rhee RY, Canton LG, McKusick MA. Surgical technique and preliminary results of endoscopic subfascial division of perforating veins. J Vasc Surg 1996; 23:517-23.

20. Iafrati MD, Welch HJ, O'Donnell TF. Subfascial endoscopic perforator ligation: An analysis of early clinical outcomes and cost. J Vasc Surg 1997; 25:995-1001.

21. Gloviczki P, Bergan JJ, Rhodes JM, Canton LG, Harmsen S, Ilstrup DM. Mid-term results of endoscopic perforator vein interruption for chronic venous insufficiency: Lessons learned from the North American Subfascial Endoscopic Perforator Surgery registry. J Vasc Surg 1999; 29:489-502.

22. Dion Y-M, Karkhouda N, Rouleau C, Audoin A. Laparoscopy-assisted aortobifemoral bypass. Surg Laparoscop Endoscop 1993: 3: 425-9.

23. Berens ES, Herde JR. Laparoscopic vascular surgery: four case reports. J Vasc Surg 1995; 22:73-9.

24. Jones DB, Thompson RW, Soper NJ, Olin JM, and Rubin BG. Development and comparison of transperitoneal and retroperitoneal approaches to laparoscopic-assisted aortofemoral bypass in a porcine model. J Vasc Surg 1996; 23:466-71.

25. Ahn SS, Hiyama DT, Rudkin GH, Fuchs GJ, Ro KM, Concepcion B. Laparoscopic aortobifemoral bypass. J Vasc Surg 1997; 26:128-32.

26. Dion Y-M, Garcia CR. A new technique for laparoscopic aortobifemoral grafting in occlusive aortoiliac disease. J Vasc Surg 1997; 26:685-92.

27. Arous EJ, Nelson PR, Yood SM, Kelly JJ, Sandor A, Litwin DEM. Hand-assisted laparoscopic aortobifemoral bypass grafting. J Vasc Surg 2000; 31:1142-8.

28. Chen MHM, D'Angelo AJ, Murphy EA, Cohen JR. laparoscopically assisted abdominal aortic aneurysm repair: a report of 10 cases. Surg Endoscopy 199: 13:77-9.

29. Kline RG, D' Angelo AJ, Chen MH, Halpern VJ, Cohen JR. Laparoscopically assisted abdominal aortic aneurysm repair: first 20 cases. J Vasc Surg 1998; 27:81-7.

30. Edoga JK, Asgarian K, Singh D, James KV, Romanelli J, Merchant S, et al. Laparoscopic surgery for abdominal aortic aneurysms: technical elements of the procedure and a preliminary report of the first 22 patients. Surg Endoscopy 1998; 12:1064-72.

31. Jobe BA, Duncan W, Swanstrom LL. Totally laparoscopic abdominal aortic aneurysm repair. Surg Endoscopy 1999; 13:77-9.

32. Kolvenbach R, Cheshire N, Pinter L, Da Silva L, Deling O, Kasper AS. Laparoscopy-assisted aneurysm resection as a minimal invasive alternative in patients unsuitable for endovascular surgery. J Vasc Surg 2001; 34:216-21.

33. Dion Y-M, Garcia CR, El Kadi HB. Totally laparoscopic abdominal aortic aneurysm repair. J Vasc Surg 2001; 33:181-5.

34. Chang DW, Chan A, Forse RA, Abbott WM. Enabling sutureless vascular bypass grafting with the exovascular sleeve anastomosis. J Vasc Surg 2000; 32:524-30.

35. Baxendale BR, Baker DM, Hutchinson A, Chuter TAM, Wenham PW, Hopkinson BR. Hemodynamic and metabolic response to endovascular repair of infra-renal aortic aneurysms. Brit J of Anesthesia 1996; 77:581-5.

36. Zarins CK, White RA, Schwarten D, Kinney E, Dietrch EB, Hodgson KJ, and Fogarty TJ. AneuRx stent graft versus open surgical repair of abdominal aortic aneurysms: multicenter prospective clinical trial. J Vasc Surg 1999; 29:292-308.

37. Moore WS, Brewster DC, Bernhard VM, for the EVT/Guidant Investigators. Aorto-uni-iliac endograft for complex aortoiliac aneurysms compared with tube/bifurcation endografts: Results of the EVT/Guidant trials. J Vasc Surg 2001; 33:S11-20.

38. Zarins CK, White RA, Moll FL, Crabtree T, Bloch DA, et al. The AneuRx stent graft: four-year results and worldwide experience 2000. J Vasc Surg 2001; 33 (2 Suppl): S135-45.

39. Anderson JL, Berce M, Hartley DE. Endoluminal aortic grafting with renal and superior mesenteric artery incorporation by graft fenestration. J Endovasc Ther 2001; 8:3-15.

40. Stanley BM, Semmens JB, Lawrence-Brown MMD, Goodman MA, Hartley DE. Fenestration in endovascular grafts for aortic aneurysm repair: new horizons for preserving blood flow in branch vessels. J Endovasc Ther 2001: 8:16-24.

41. Chuter TAM, Gordon RL, Reilly LM, Goodman JD, Messina LM. An endovascular system for thoracoabdominal aortic aneurysm repair. J Endovasc Ther 2001; 8:25-33.

42. Chuter TAM, Gordon RL, Reilly LM, Pak LK, Messina LM. Multi-branched stent-graft for type III thoracoabdominal aortic aneurysm. J Vasc Intervent Radiol 2001:12: 391-2.

43. Ohki T, Veith FJ, Sanchez LA, Cynamon J, Lipsitz EC, et al. Endovascular graft repair of ruptured aortoiliac aneurysms. J Am Coll Surg 1999; 189: 102-13.

44. Greenberg RK, Srivastava SD, Ouriel K, Waldman D, Ivancev K, et al. An endoluminal method of hemorrhage control and repair of ruptured abdominal aortic aneurysms. J Endovasc Ther 2000; 7:1-7.

45. Rici MA, Knight SJ, Nutter B, Callas PW. Desktop telemedicine in vascular surgery: some preliminary findings. Telemedicine J 1998; 4:279-85.

46. Bowersox JC. Telepresence surgery. Brit J Surg 1996; 83:433-4.

47. Bowersox JC, Shah A, Jensen J, Hill J, Cordts PR, Green PS. Vascular applications of telepresence surgery: initial feasibility studies in swine. J Vasc Surg 1996; 23:281-7.

48. Li R, Jensen J, Hill J, Bowersox JC. Quantitative evaluation of surgical task performance by remote-access endoscopic telemanipulation. Surg Endoscopy 2000; 14:431-5.

49. Li RA, Jensen J, Bowersox JC. Microvascular anastomoses performed in rats using a microsurgical telemanipulator. Computer Aided Surg 2000; 5:326-32.

50. Boehm DH, Reichenspurner H, Detter C, Arnold M, Gulbins H, et al. Clinical use of a computer-enhanced surgical robotic system for endoscopic coronary artery bypass grafting in the beating heart. Thor Cardiovasc Surg 2000; 48:198-202.

51. Calligaro KD, Dougherty MJ, Patterson DE, Raviola CA, DeLaurentis DA. Value of an endovascular suite in the operating room. Ann of Vasc Surg 1998; 12:296-8.

52. Mansour MA, Hodgson KF. Preparing the endovascular operating room suite. In Moore WS and Ahn SS (eds): Endovascular Surgery. Philadelphia, PA, W.B. Saunders Company, 2001, pp. 3-13.

53. Mansour MA. The new operating room environment. Surg Clin North America 1999; 79:477-87.

54. Zarins CK. Presidential address: Time for the future of Vascular Surgery. J Vasc Surg 2000; 31:207-16.

CHAPTER 17

THE ECONOMICS OF HEALTH CARE

PAUL A. TAHERI, M.D., M.B.A.

Introduction

Health care is changing as rapidly as technology advances. Over the past decade, we have experienced tumultuous, technology-driven change in the financing, economics, and delivery of care. This continuous change shows no signs of abating.

The "cost-plus" and "fee-for-service" 1970s are now recognized as the "golden era" of American medicine. Physicians ruled the health care landscape. Incomes were high, their authority unquestioned, and their prestige unparalleled. However, this prized status declined steadily over the ensuing decades, eroded by ever escalating costs, growing societal pressures, and perceived inefficiencies in the delivery of care. These and many other issues ushered in a decade of cost containment, new insurance instruments – collectively referred to as "managed care" – and the introduction of "gatekeepers" and other institutional "innovations" designed to actively manage all aspects of the patients' disease. Physicians often interpreted managed care to mean "rationed care," and in practice much of managed care has indeed been devoted to reducing resource consumption patient by patient.

The 1980s and the early 1990s were characterized by health system overcapacity and unimpeded access to tertiary facilities. Hospitals, health systems, and physicians aggressively signed contracts even when those contracts reimbursed less than total cost. Facing shrinking (and often negative) margins, the industry consolidated; hospitals either closed or merged into larger provider networks. These market forces drove many physician specialists from their solo or hospital-based practices into large, independent physician groups. Many primary care physicians had their practices acquired by health systems intent on assuring themselves of a steady flow into their core inpatient businesses irrespective of the underlying economic logic.

Since the mid-1990s, health care has been in a state of flux, as the surfeit of hospital capacity evaporated – both because of a reduction in hospital "beds" (more than1000 hospitals have closed in the U.S. in recent years) and a sharp, unanticipated increase in demand. Nationwide hospital occupancy rates have risen swiftly and to the point that even from a financial perspective congestion costs often outweigh any advantages that might result from higher throughput and more fully amortized overhead. (See the rising unit costs illustrated for a hypothetical inpatient procedure Figure 1). Patients routinely suffer the inconveniences of long queues, and increasingly these delays affect the quality of care for patients who simply can not wait. Care has been compromised.

Academic health systems face unique responsibilities and thus special circumstances. They have been more adversely affected than other health systems by the difficult financial environment, in no small part because they function at a greater scale and scope than other providers. Given the complexities of care at academic health systems, and the attendant financial risks, their financial targets looking forward seem modest, at best. The University of Michigan Health System, for example, aims for just a two percent operating margin on an annual clinical revenue stream exceeding $1 billion.

Shifting Market Forces

Capacity reductions have combined with a marked increase in technology- and demographics-induced demand to create an abrupt reversal of the economic forces shaping health care. A November 2001 study, The New Economics of Care, the Advisory Board reaches a variety of conclusions about trends in health care economics that it says, "... may prove as wrenching to hospitals as the transition from fee-for-service to managed care a decade ago." Specifically, it reports that "... in just the last year or so, all signs point to a sea change in hospital supply and demand; to the mind

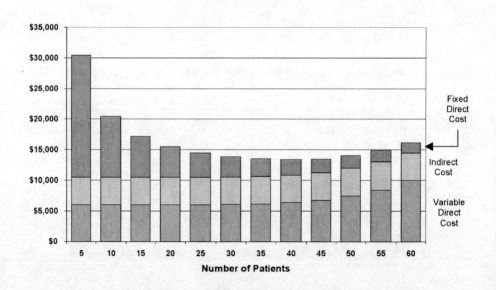

Figure 17-1
Relationship between total cost and patient volumes.
VDC = Variable direct costs;
IC = Indirect costs; FDC = Fixed direct costs.

of some, hospitals [are] rapidly exiting an era of surplus, and entering a period of prolonged and chronic shortage." The study also concludes that medical admissions are growing much faster than surgical admissions, claiming a greater share of available capacity, and in many cases surgical admissions are being crowded out. These same conclusions are echoed by other sources, including The New York Times (e.g., "Patients Surge and Hospitals Hunt for Beds," March 28, 2002).

Managing for throughput optimization requires an in-depth analysis of the process for care delivery. Understanding the fundamental economics of hospital-based care is critical to optimizing the clinical delivery of care. Specifically, hospitals have a high fixed cost and low marginal cost associated with the delivery of care. From a clinician perspective, the bulk of each health care dollar goes to the "overhead" associated with the delivery of care (the sum of fixed direct and indirect costs). More specifically, studies have demonstrated that this "overhead" can be as high as 85% in the very short run (when even inputs such as nursing are largely fixed) and 65% in the longer run. The remaining "variable costs" stem from the actual delivery of care to individual patients. These are the only hospital expenses under physicians' direct and immediate control.

As the aforementioned curve identifies, the more patients "pushed" through the system, the lower the fixed costs associated with the delivery of care. However, at some point this amortization of costs reaches a nadir and the cost begins to rise, and at some point to escalate rapidly. Thus the right side of this U-shaped curve demonstrates the costs associated with congestion, or over subscription of care or from an economics perspective, where demand outstrips capacity.

Capacity Shortages Generate New System Issues

Once capacity becomes congested, or oversubscribed, it is important to consider the "opportunity cost" of each new admission. Providers must identify what each admission means in terms of opportunities forgone. Providers that are filling their beds with patients who do not support the hospital's mission (whether this is research, teaching, service, profit, or all of the above) must ask the question of which patients, procedures, activities, and programs they should be supporting. Health systems that are unable to bring in high margin business are seeing a recently described phenomenon of "profitless growth."

These capacity trends and the attendant sequale are especially ominous for academic health systems for several reasons. First and foremost, the uncertainty and high variability attending complex care will have more adverse consequences than in the past, when hospitals operated with fewer bottlenecks and spare capacity. Disruptions attributable to the emergent and complex service will grow more frequent and more problematic; wait times will increase throughout academic health systems and hospitals will be forced to invest more to coordinate care and to expand capacity. Second, and related, hospitals face higher opportunity costs of providing highly variable critical care, meaning that with capacity constrained they face more serious tradeoffs between providing disruptive emergent complex care and pursuing other more profitable clinical activities.

Understanding the economics of care delivery is central to developing a credible plan for transforming that delivery. While health systems are accumulating greater institutional capabilities to increase throughput – to dispense more care with the same fixed resource – doing so requires credible (and often complex) implementation plans that are both accepted and driven by physicians. The key to success is "buy-in" from clinicians. Administrative fiat, regulatory mandate, and payer pressure can all materially influence delivery; and yet none of these models is ultimately as effective as a focused implementation strategy that includes active physician input. Creating an environment for system change can only be achieved through understanding the current structure of the physician relationship within the health system.

Silos as Barriers to Implementation

Most health systems are organized into clinical departments. As such, many aspects of care are weighed down by a clinically oriented "silo" mentality, which can manifest itself in multiple domains as diverse as, say, the recruitment of physicians and unwarranted attachments to legacy computer systems. Yet silo effects may be most evident in the lack of coordination of individual patients' care. Understanding the care pathway for elective services (hip arthoplasty, coronary artery bypass surgery, or a hernia repair) is characterized by unique and variable bottlenecks in scheduling, physician availability, bed allocations, and test result verification. Collectively, these activities cause an appearance of a system that is non-communicative, redundant, inefficient, and Byzantine.

Even above the operational level, lack of coordination is often evident. From a strategic planning perspective, most departments hire new faculty based upon their own narrow clinical or research needs, while the hospital, knowing little or nothing about this recruit, may be ill-equipped to handle the demand for services that this individual or department has generated. Hiring a new cardiac surgeon, for example, creates demands on the system that may already be maximally taxed such as, requiring more operating room capacity, perfusion technology, and clinic space.

How Should We Proceed?

As we enter an era of capacity constraints – with bottlenecks in both facilities and human resources – how should we modify the way we deliver patient care? What tools do we need to proceed? In certain respects, we must not change at all. We must continue to hold the physician-patient relationship sacrosanct, and advocate aggressively and effectively on our patients' behalves. We must resist unwarranted efforts to ration fixed capacity, just as in the past we successfully resisted managed care rules that sought merely to ration those variable resources that our patients needed. And whatever reasonable measures we adopt to manage scarce capacity, they must emanate from a well-reasoned perspective that derives directly and immediately from the core transaction between a physician and patient. Whether it is the hospital information technology infrastructure, radiology services, operating room facilities, billing procedures, health system contracting, utilization review processes, or risk management programs, innovation must proceed within the context of individual physicians representing the best interests of their individual patients.

To succeed at reforming their health systems while also representing both their individual patients (first) and their individual departments (thereafter), all physicians must gain at least a rudimentary understanding of the managerial underpinnings of health care. They must i) come to grips with such terms as marginal cost, opportunity cost, overhead, throughput, risk management, and capital budgeting; ii) they must insist on the requisite data (timely, accurate, complete, ...) to apply these concepts to their own health systems; and iii) they must learn and deploy strong leadership skills, and enlist others to join in the effort. This last step requires, among other measures, that physicians and administrators work together to rethink and realign incentives, and to credibly commit to them. Unfortunately, while physicians are increasingly being asked/required to become more active and engaged in managing their health system, few physicians have any formal management training, or any reliable data, or the leadership opportunities or incentives to succeed.

The growing ranks of physician leaders who administer large clinical domains unfortunately lack the basic skill set to manage effectively. They are set up to fail, or at least to do no better than muddle along by virtue of sheer will and hard work. Throughout their many years of undergraduate and graduate coursework, their residencies, their continuing medical education, and their long professional careers, they rarely, if ever, have the opportunity to learn the basics of economics, cost accounting, risk management, finance and financial accounting, or operations management. Clinical expertise and good health system management are essential to the sustained viability of a health system. In addition to the dearth of physician management skills, physicians are often shut out of health systems' strategic planning, and they are typically denied adequate data to optimize even their own units' performance. At best, they receive months-old summary statistics on average margins and cost per case, with no detail on outliers, cost drivers, or other underlying determinants of cost-effectiveness.

Yet these same physicians are more and more often held accountable for the costs of patient care, and the primitive levers they have historically used to manage costs have proven ineffective. Thus, for example, hospital-based physicians are often judged according to their patients' average length of stay (LOS), and yet two decades of LOS reductions have both failed to stem the steady rise in health care costs and left little room for further gains. Moreover, evidence is mounting that LOS was all along a misguided metric: patients who are sicker cost more on average and stay in the hospital longer, but the correlation between cost and LOS is almost entirely spurious. Lopping days off the ends of patients' stays accomplishes far less than physicians have been led to believe – unless, of course, doing so frees up capacity that will then be used to treat more patients. More generally, many physicians no longer consider LOS and other crude metrics credible, and increasingly they ignore administrators who measure their performance in these terms.

Despite their lack of formal training, many physicians have significant administrative responsibilities, and they want to perform well. They recognize that the financial stakes are often huge, and increasingly they reject a reigning health care paradigm that assumes a fundamental conflict between financial and clinical success. They want to manage their patients' care rather than simply ration it.

Understanding how to manage requires a new level of commitment from both the organization and the clinician. Health systems must provide the opportunity to educate and integrate physician administrators into the health system matrix, and physicians must take the time to develop their managerial skill set. The future of health care is bright and the management of this industry should rest with the physician leader.

CHAPTER 18

THE OR OF THE FUTURE: BILLING AND DOCUMENTATION

RONALD B. HIRSCHL, M.D.

In the current medical economic climate, surgeons are performing more operations with lower reimbursement and increasing administrative overhead. This is unlikely to change. Limited budgets will drive Medicare and Medicaid, as well as commercial insurers, managed care, and other insurance companies, to decrease costs and to increase regulations in an already complex system in order to further reduce payment. Surgeons, in turn, must adapt and use innovative means to win this Darwinian struggle with payers. The purpose of this discussion will be to speculate on how that adaptation and innovation will look to the surgeon of the 21st Century.

The initial premise is that paper will become obsolete. At the University of Michigan, we have developed the Surgery Tracking and Reporting application (STAR), also known as Clinical Charge Capture (C3), which has completely removed paper from the preauthorization, charge capture, coding, review, and documentation process (See Figures 1 and 2). With this system, preauthorization for specific Common Procedure Terminology (CPT) and International Classification of Diagnoses (ICD-9) codes is documented online prior to performance of a procedure. At the time of a procedure, these codes can be used to seamlessly bill for what was preauthorized or the physician can capture a charge and initiate coding using a variety of user-friendly approaches, including keyword searches, organization of procedures by organ systems, and development of personal libraries. It is likely that such charge capture and coding will be performed in the operating room in the future by voice recognition, via extraction from documentation by other caretakers, and/or by word recognition from dictated documentation. Otherwise, wireless, handheld computing device, laptops, personal digital assistants (PDAs), or web pads (portable laptop-sized devices with touch sensitive screens) will be used to capture charges in a mobile environment. These devices will allow charge capture in the operating room, on the floors, and in the clinics during performance of patient care and consult services as well as following minor and major procedures.

With the current system at the University of Michigan, captured and coded charges are reviewed online by billing specialists before being sent to clearinghouses, which act as intermediaries for bill distribution and reimbursement, or directly to payers. This manual review process will likely disappear as the rules for billing are incorporated into charge capture and review software applications. Once reviewed, charges will be sent directly to payers: clearinghouses will fade away as the direct links between providers and payers removes the need for these costly intermediaries in the billing process. Currently, the STAR/C3 system allows surgeons to receive and analyze online payments and rejections received by the clearinghouse. As the direct link between the surgeon's practice and the payers is developed, reimbursement will become automated so that payments will be sent and directly received by much more efficient, organized, and less complex methods.

The paper form of documentation will disappear. Dictation will be conducted via handheld, mobile devices and will reside in digital form. At the University of Michigan, all operative documentation is processed online by the STAR/C3 system. Notes which are generated from templates or transcribed from digital telephone dictation systems are edited and signed online at the same time that attestation with regard to presence of the teaching physician are appended. Within the next 5 to 10 years, voice recognition systems will become refined, routinely available, and widely applied. It is likely that surgeons will dictate via headsets in the operating room with an operative note completed and available for editing by "transcriptionists" or by the surgeon at the completion of a procedure. Templates, with targeted drop down menus to cover areas of typical variation in a procedure, will be the norm and will be available to provide documentation for all but the most unusual procedures. Perhaps digital documentation will never even be transcribed into a "readable" document. For instance, documentation may take the form of a digital video which demonstrates the procedure performed and even the presence of the surgeon in doing so. Perhaps audio files of operative dictations will be saved digitally, rather than being transcribed. In one form or another, multimedia documentation will be available online to other physicians and insurance companies for both patient care, billing, and reimbursement purposes. As with the current STAR/C3 billing process, these automated systems which incorporate online documentation will better allow the surgeon to support billing claims and to counter rejections of bills by payers.

It is likely and appropriate that the current complex, confusing, disorganized, archaic, and unstandardized billing system will be revised. Legislation to encourage and even to enforce timely and accurate payment will begin to bring fair business practices to the healthcare industry. Hospitals, consumers, and the healthcare industry, perhaps in conjunction with the state and federal Legislatures, will push to standardize and markedly reduce the complexity of billing, coding, and even reimbursement rules and processes. Insurance companies will be more closely linked in the digital world with physicians. Although payers tend to shun automated bill submission and payment, since chaos and inefficiency result in decreased charges and payment, automated, efficient links between surgeons and payers will prevail because of the reduction in costs associated with better organization, fewer billing errors, and decreased manual processes. Pre-authorization for procedures will either not be required with this standardized process or will be obtained online via integration of systems between the surgeon's practice and the payer.

All of this, of course, will depend on the healthcare reimbursement process which we have in the United States. Will we have a national health plan? Will we continue to have both private and state/federal reimbursement for healthcare? Will managed care and health maintenance organizations continue to be a major force in the healthcare marketplace? How we bill and document will depend on the payer landscape and legislation which will change what is required in the charge capture, coding, compliance, and documentation process. Whatever that process, it is certain that the charge capture, billing, documentation, and reimbursement system will be automated. We no longer can afford to have inefficient, disorganized, incomplete, and inaccurate billing systems. Thus, applications which automate the billing and documentation process will be widely used to enhance the ability of the surgeon to fairly and appropriately be compensated for the skill, work, and risks associated with the performance of procedures both in and out of the operating room.

CHAPTER 19

ANESTHESIA INFORMATION SYSTEMS

MICHAEL O'REILLY, M.D., M.S. AND KEVIN K. TREMPER, M.D., PH.D

One of the greatest challenges facing physicians in the 21st century is information management. The unaided human mind cannot keep up with the results of clinical trials, the ever changing government regulations or the introduction of new drugs, techniques and devices. For example, between 1966 and 1995 the number of randomized controlled trials in the USA increased from 100 to 10,000 per year.(1) Without question we must apply computers and information systems to integrate new information and knowledge into our practice for the sake of our patients, our health systems and our professional well-being.

Anesthesiologists face many of the same problems as practitioners in other specialties and have the additional challenge, and opportunity, of using many different computers in the course of their everyday activities. However, in spite of the explosion in the use of computers and information systems in virtually every industry much medical information is still managed using a paper and pen. Physiologic monitors are specialized computers and anesthesia machines, gas analyzers and infusion pumps all contain computers of one sort or another. The opportunity to integrate the information they generate provides exciting opportunities to make our jobs easier while providing safer and more efficient care for our patients and our health systems.

The Paper Based System Has Got to Go

Information is essential to the management of any business, and the business of medicine is an information intensive business. Could you imagine what it would be like if you went to your bank to see if a recent deposit had been credited to your account and they told you to have a seat while they sent for your records? "Oh, you made the deposit at a different branch? Make yourself comfortable while we send for those records. Are you sure it was a $1,000 deposit?" Would it make you more comfortable if four different people asked you that same question "Was it $1,000"? While many of us may hold our health as dear as our money, the information infrastructure for health care is primitive and much of the information we use is still stored on paper. This is a problem for several reasons but mostly because the patients now move through the system faster than their paper charts. Thus it so often happens that, the patient arrives in the operating room one day after being seen in the clinic and the chart is still in the clinic. Another major problem with the current paper based system is that multiple people need the same information at the same time in different places. Our clinics and health systems are continually growing and separating geographically. Different specialists and technicians are likely to be involved with a patient's care at the same time. All relevant caregivers need access to patient information at many times and many sites. Other businesses have solved this problem. Our patients may get asked five times or more if they have allergies to medicines. We rationalize this redundant questioning by assuming "it gives them confidence in our thoroughness." If you went to a hotel and they asked your name five times would you think they were being thorough or just a bunch of idiots? When patients report for an operative procedure they are likely to become quite anxious when asked the same question repeatedly. Such anxiety may translate, for example, into concern for our ability to have all the right parts for their total hip. So we sedate them (we anesthesiologists have drugs). Clearly, we need point of care information in real time. Although no one using paper charts needs a study to prove that paperbased systems are flawed, one study did confirm that paper charts are not always delivered when and where they are needed.(2)

Information Systems Will Help Us Practice Evidence Based Medicine

Information systems will help us practice evidence based medicine in two ways. First, for instances with clear and convincing evidence that care should be delivered with a particular combination of drugs and techniques, the information system will integrate the practice guidelines with clinical documentation. At the University of Michigan we do this with the use of "case-based defaults." The case-based defaults are the series of actions taken by the anesthesiologist in the course of delivering an anesthetic and they are presented as a script in the order that things are done. As the script is followed, the care provided is documented and the provider is prompted to do the right thing, i.e. follow the protocol. The reasons for deviations from the script (practice guidelines) can be used to refine the script further and validate its effectiveness. For example, if someone deviates from the script because the patient has a particular comorbidity, say hypertension, we can then go back and analyze the outcomes for patients with hypertension where the script was followed and determine whether that particular deviation had a beneficial effect. In addition, justifiable deviations from the script may be based on educational or research objectives. In those cases we will be able to quantify the additional costs associated with those missions. Information systems will also help in those cases without clear consensus regarding the optimal combination of drugs and techniques. Here patients can be randomized to one of two or more practice guidelines (scripts). In this manner every patient is either part of the study group or part of the control group, thus creating a continuous feedback loop to provide additional evidence to improve practice guidelines. Deficiencies in study design will be compensated by the large number of cases we can efficiently capture and analyze. These data can be translated into information and knowledge that parlays into clinical practice.

Health Care is Changing

There has been a fundamental shift in the forces that affect health care delivery. Cost must be balanced with risk and benefit as we determine the best way to treat patients: Surgical services typically generate about half of most hospitals' revenue and consume about half the resources. Anesthesiology potentially has a large impact on health systems. Information systems will close the disconnects between what we do, how the patients react, and how satisfied the patients are with their care. In business terms, "If you can't measure it you can't manage it." Cost data integrated with the case based defaults/practice guidelines described above will necessitate consideration of the tradeoffs involving differences in cost, outcome and patient satisfaction. What cost justifies improved patient satisfaction?

Anesthesiologists are the Co-morbidity and Phenotype Doctors

Besides putting patients to sleep and waking them up, the practice of anesthesiology consists of identifying and optimizing a patient's comorbidities. Comorbidity identification of has critical implications because many payers base reimbursement on the Diagnosis Related Group (DRG) system. The DRG classification changes based on whether or not patients have comorbidities or complications and accurate anesthesia comorbidity documentation increases DRG based reimbursement from 1.5 to 5%.(3, 4) Our own studies at the University of Michigan measuring the impact of anesthesiology comorbidity capture have found a similar favorable effect.

In addition, our quality assurance program seeks to capture all perioperative complications and we expect this too will impact DRG reimbursements. A further step to increase the capture of comorbidities will be to employ logic and reminders. In the case of comorbidities, the patient may take medications or have lab or other test results that suggest a diagnosis. For example, if the patient is taking synthroid, the preoperative history and physical will not let you complete "normal" for the endocrine system without acknowledging a prompt that says "patient is on synthroid, is hypothyroidism documented?" Similarly for a patient has a low hematocrit following surgery, the system will prompt blood loss anemia, a commonly missed complication. If a patient has an elevated troponin following surgery the practitioner will be queried if the patient had a myocardial infarction. Implementing the logic is straightforward; modifying all the other associated processes will be the challenge.

As the human genome is elucidated we will want to correlate genotype with phenotype. There will be the opportunity for a convergence of bioinformatics with clinical informatics to fundamentally alter the way we deliver drugs. We will be able to watch and measure how patients respond to drugs in real time. It is likely that we will be able to predict how an individual patient will respond to a particular drug or combination of drugs, so as to tailor an anesthetic specific for an individual's genetics. This will be a significant improvement over our current "titrate to effect" approach.

Information Systems Will Improve Patient Safety

As pointed out in the recent Institute of Medicine report about patient safety, information systems hold great promise for optimizing patient safety.(5) Since anesthesiologists use many different physiologic monitors that are essentially computers, we have a great opportunity to leverage their integration and improve safety. We consistently see near misses that could have been detected earlier if simple logic had been applied to the available information. For example, if the pulse oximeter loses the signal and at the same time there is a precipitous drop in the end-tidal carbon dioxide, a patient has had a potentially catastrophic drop in cardiac output. We need to employ the same methodologies of the airline and nuclear power plant industries to the operating room and other critical care environments to have the equivalent of the "pull up, pull up" alert that prevents pilot from flying into mountains. In anesthesiologic forms this would prevent us from moving the pulse oximeter from finger to finger only to be told by the surgeon "the blood is looking awful dark down here."

Information Systems Will Make Our Jobs Easier

Most initial efforts to "computerize" anesthesia documentation centered on a computerized anesthesia record. Since the monitors had ports, enterprising anesthesiologists wrote computer programs that would capture blood pressure and heart rate into nicely documented anesthesia records.(6, 7) Computerized anesthesia records offer limited added value because paper records and pens are cheap. More useful to the anesthesiologist are tools that improve the perioperative workflow so that the right information is available at the point of care. For example, many cases are expensively delayed in the OR because the patient informed consent cannot be located. Systems that reduce delays, for lack of signed consent or history and physical, offer value to all the stakeholders (hospital, surgeons, nurses and anesthesiologist). Another vexing problem, particularly for an institution taking care of complex patients is ensuring proper follow up for test results. Patients coming to the Patient Advanced Testing clinic may require a stress test prior to their surgery. The reporting of that information to the anesthesiologist who will actually be caring for the patient is problematic. An information system that is integrated with the scheduling system and includes pending work list with email and paging alerts can solve the problem.

Information Systems Will Make Us Better Teachers

In fulfilling our educational mission, the Internet and intranet allow us to provide context sensitive information to our medical students and residents while they are in the practice of actually delivering care. This ability has a dual benefit of providing ready reference material that can be applied in real time at the bedside and in enriching the educational experience by having the appropriate information available that pertains to a particular patient's condition right at the optimal moment for the trainee. Direct links to the rationale behind practice guidelines will reinforce their importance and improve compliance. For those of us who are further from our training the ability to access this information at the bedside has already shown its value.

Privacy and Information Systems

Many states have laws protecting patient privacy; however, until the passage of the Health Insurance Portability and Accountability Act Of 1996 (HIPAA) the Federal Government had no regulations governing patient privacy and security of healthcare information. With the implementation of HIPAA come a host of challenges to comply with the regulations. In addition, the Federal Medicare and Medicaid programs have specific regulations and requirements for compliance and documentation. Information systems are the only practical way to implement, enforce and monitor compliance and ensure privacy. Additional technical challenges must be addressed to ensure the computer systems are encrypted and secure but certainly they should be more secure the paper based records.

In Summary

The challenge of high quality health care delivery at low cost requires collection and analysis of information. The codification of large amounts of data allows us to make associations between what we do and how well the patients perform as a routine part of the practice. An information system can conduct this analysis more efficiently and faster than hitherto imagined. Eventually, every patient will be part of on ongoing study to improve the quality of care and service provided. As academic physicians, we must create knowledge from information. Computers and information systems are clearly the tools of the age for handling information. If we apply these tools cleverly they will make a major impact in our missions of clinical care, education, research and the fiscal bottom line. They also will improve the job satisfaction of the anesthesiologists, nurses, surgeons and others who interact in our intense and stressful critical care environments.

REFERENCES

1. Chassin MR. Is health care ready for Six Sigma quality? Milbank Quarterly 1998; 76:565-91.

2. Elson RB, Faughnan JG, Connelly DP. An industrial process view of information delivery to support clinical decision making: implications for systems design and process measures. J Am Med Inform Assoc 1997; 4:266-78.

3. Gibby GL, et. al. Increased comorbidity diagnosis and hospital reimbursement from computerized preanesthetic evaluation system. Anesthesiology 1994; 81:A1229.

4. Gibby GL, et. al. Computerized preanesthesia evaluation of surgical patients increases secondary diagnosis noted by hospital coders. J of Clin Monitoring 1995; 11:268.

5. Kohn LT, Corrigan J, Donaldson MS. To err is human : building a safer health system. Washington, D.C.: National Academy Press, 2000:xxi, 287.

6. Shaffer MJ, Kaiser PR, Klingenmaier CH, Gordon MR. Manual record-keeping and statistical records for the operating room. Med Instrum 1978; 12:192-7.

7. Reich DL, Wood RK, Jr., Mattar R, et al. Arterial blood pressure and heart rate discrepancies between handwritten and computerized anesthesia records. Anesthesia & Analgesia 2000; 91:612-6.

CHAPTER 20

SURGICAL EDUCATION

J. ROLAND FOLSE, M.D.

Stephen Hawking, the renowned physicist, in his book, The Illustrated Brief History of Time, concludes that "humanity's deepest desire for knowledge is justification enough for our continued quest". For physicians, the desire to protect and prolong life continues to push scientific discovery and methods of healing. As educators, we search for a better understanding of how we learn and how we can prolong the quest for discovery by teaching and stimulating those who will follow us. Education is more than teaching – it encompasses the leadership to build structures and faculty; it sets the background and environment to enhance learning; it defines the diversity of individual differences and it provides purpose for learning.

For many decades, medical education and particularly surgical training, was an on-the-job apprentice experience, guided by highly disciplined and motivated individuals. It was a very successful educational model because it was small, usually confined to a closed hospital setting, and driven primarily by a value system based on physician-patient relationship. Knowledge was transmitted by direct teaching or reading, and skills were developed by practice under supervision. Discipline, the driving force for excellence, was developed as a part of team interaction and competition. Just as an army squad or as a football team develops a sense of discipline by team effort, surgical trainees over a several year period developed discipline and, with it, competence and self-reliance. Bedside rounds, abundant operative experiences, and diverse outpatient clinics provided ample opportunities for seeing, doing and learning. In general, the hospital environment welcomed the student and trainee as a necessary part of the patient care team and the trainees immersed themselves, night and day, into the learning and healing environment with little personal financial reward and little concern about a life outside the hospital. Learning was successful because it was repetitious, it was practice oriented, and because mentors, faculty or upper level residents, provided instruction and feedback. It is worth remembering that those who entered the medical field were uniquely driven, accepted the rigors of the experience as a rite of passage, and often planned for medicine to be their one calling in life. In short, traditional medical and surgical training, until the last two decades, was a reflection of the mores of the individuals and the environment where training took place.

Everyone, those within and without the medical profession, is aware of the major impact that changes in health care delivery have had in the medical profession – and very significantly on medical education. This impact on education, brought about by changes in health finances, patient education and involvement and the newer ambulatory sites for delivery, has been a wake up call for those who are responsible for educating future physicians and ensuring that good patient care continues to be paramount. No longer can leisurely bed side teaching take place; no longer can residents independently conduct operative procedures; no longer will residents be expected to work both day and night, even at the expense of loss of continuity of care; and no longer will surgery departments be ivory towers of research with practice as a secondary endeavor.

Even with the unforeseen changes brought about by health care reform, it is gratifying to see the responses of the educational community to adjust and to improve its quality of education and to refocus the important issues necessary to maintain a great profession.

Undergraduate medical education is in a process of evolution. Many medical students are adopting different approaches to the pathways to becoming a physician. Small group discussions have replaced many lectures and performance is judged equally as important as knowledge. Many schools are attempting to merge the basic sciences with clinical medicine by introducing relevant clinical experiences into the first two years of medical school. Problem-based learning focuses on real patient problems where students in small groups with a tutor explore basic science issues in a clinical context and develop skills of inquiry, interaction, and integration. The use of the internet and new technologies are, and will more in the future, greatly facilitating the immediacy of finding answers and applying them to clinical solutions. Many institutions have developed educational resource centers where simulated patient encounters take place in a clinical setting with an instructor and classmates observing and participating. With the rapidly expanding body of knowledge and the availability of new developments, all students must develop the tools to be self-directed, lifelong learners. The evaluation of these skills requires more than paper and pencil testing. Performance based evaluation, now standard in Canadian licensure exams, will be used more and more to evaluate students, residents, and practicing physicians. Simulated clinical problems using actor patients have been extensively studied and validated and will be combined with computer simulations and virtual reality to measure performance. All medical schools are adapting to the new clinical environment and practice guidelines. Unfortunately, the place of medical students in the new setting has not been given a primary focus. It will require innovation to maintain student-patient interaction in the new health care environment, but they must not be excluded.

Recently, graduate medical education has expanded its focus and requirements to include new competencies. This is a long needed readjustment in priorities, for it emphasizes such important concepts as learning from and improving practice, improving interpersonal and communication skills, developing ethical and professional stature and organizing system-based practices. Already the residency review committees and the specialty boards have adopted guidelines for implementation of these concepts. As programs develop blueprints for incorporating their competencies into training, it will be important that the methods used are educationally sound, can be studied and validated, and will have outcome measures. It is not enough to lay out ethical concepts or practice management seminars without providing a means to make them a daily way of life.

Surgical training programs face major educational hurdles in the future. A shortened work schedule in the face of rapidly advancing new technology and a mandate to document competency, makes the traditional approach to teaching and learning difficult or impossible.

One solution being studied by several institutions is the use of surgical skills labs. It was the onset of laparoscopic surgery that stimulated the development of skills laboratories, but many are going beyond these technologies. The use of a simulation or practice lab to acquire technical skills before applying them to actual patients not only may reduce errors but may be more cost efficient. Some lab procedures not only provide practice, but also insert decision-making, error prevention, and new encounters into the sessions. Labs are expensive to set up, but if they are integrated into the training program and used extensively, there actually may be a savings in overall cost. Other professions are certainly more advanced in the use of simulation than the medical profession and much can be learned from existing technology. A better understanding of the stages of automated expertise development has allowed the process of developing and practicing a skill to be broken down into components in order to study and control development in the various stages. By moving part of the learning curve out of the OR, junior residents are more efficient and safer when they accept responsibility for performance on patients. Many prerequisite skills for students and junior residents can be broken down into components, some learned on models, some on the computer, and some in a lab with monitoring and controls. Practice in the lab allows for attainment of the skills at the appropriate level by repetition and correction of errors with formative feedback.

One of the greatest challenges finishing surgical trainees face is how they will maintain competence throughout a surgical career. One of the hallmarks of a professional is continuing education and maintenance of competency, yet organized medicine has generally provided only basic knowledge updates from journals and conferences. After residency, the opportunities for acquiring new skills are limited, although hands-on courses such as for ultrasound, breast biopsy, and sentinel node mapping are developing. It will be important that such courses not only provide instruction but provide practice under surveillance and long term follow-up. The American College of Surgeons and other national surgical organizations should take a lead in setting standards for such courses by providing the educational framework that will allow consistency among medical institutions and hospitals, likely to become the schools for new technology courses.

The issue of continued certification of competency is receiving much discussion, but the tools and the organizations for this are not settled. The career pathways of most surgeons are quite variable depending upon location and changing personal opportunities or interests. Yet, regardless of extent or content of a surgical practice, it must be competently performed. First and foremost, it is important that the physician desires to maintain an up-to-date practice and has the personal skills and the opportunities to continue to progress. Support by local colleagues and institutions is paramount and facilities should be developed to allow extended skills training on a regional basis. Medical schools and teaching hospitals are the logical sites to provide such continued training. It will be important for the medical and surgical supply industry to set aside parochial interests and participate in this general, ongoing education. The internet provides an accessible, daily opportunity to get immediate answers to medical questions. It may be the single, most efficient means for problem solving for the physician. Already students and residents are using on-line sources for daily patient care questions and as an extension of printed texts and journals.

Research in medical education is quite extensive, much of it devoted to teaching, curricular development and evaluation; yet, surgical education, particularly intra-operative technical education, has not been as well studied. Educational research is clear in defining the teaching qualities that are most effective – objectivity and support instead of intimidation, a mentor or coach instead of a platoon leader. Sometimes surgeons who are decisive and quick in the trauma room carry hurried attitudes into teaching sessions. Utmost concern for patient care and safety can be a barrier to effective teaching unless surgeons are able to consciously separate the needs of the patient and the needs of the learner. Residents have so closely integrated their patient care and learning that they often neglect their personal life. New research is urgently needed to study the impacts of shorter work hours, breaks in continuity of care, laboratory based learning, performance evaluation, and maintaining continuing competence.

Many younger academic surgeons are spending time studying surgical teaching and devoting their research careers to educational issues. Challenges extend from developing better individual teachers to finding solutions to how new procedures and technologies can be smoothly incorporated into surgical practice. Surgeons must develop methods of assessment which look past knowledge evaluation to skills, practice, and communication. Simulators, role playing, virtual reality, and the internet require more research and development. Yet, no new device or technique will replace the teacher who can stimulate new learning and inspire stellar performance. Teaching is a learned skill, not often an innate trait, but a skill all surgeons should possess as proficiently as their operative skills.

INDEX